STUDY GUIDE TO NEUROPSYCHIATRY AND BEHAVIORAL NEUROSCIENCES

A Companion to
The American Psychiatric Publishing
Textbook of Neuropsychiatry
and Behavioral Neurosciences,
Fifth Edition

STUDY GUIDE TO NEUROPSYCHIATRY AND BEHAVIORAL NEUROSCIENCES

A Companion to The American Psychiatric Publishing Textbook of Neuropsychiatry and Behavioral Neurosciences, Fifth Edition

Robert E. Hales, M.D.
Joe P. Tupin Professor and Chair
Department of Psychiatry and Behavioral Sciences
University of California, Davis
School of Medicine
Sacramento, California

James A. Bourgeois, O.D., M.D.
Alan Stoudemire Professor of Psychosomatic Medicine
Department of Psychiatry and Behavioral Sciences
University of California, Davis Medical Center
School of Medicine
Sacramento, California

Narriman C. Shahrokh
Chief Administrative Officer
Department of Psychiatry and Behavioral Sciences
University of California, Davis
School of Medicine
Sacramento, California

American Psychiatric Publishing, Inc.
Washington, DC
London, England

Manufactured in the United States of America on acid-free paper
11 10 09 08 07 5 4 3 2 1

ISBN-13 978-1-58562-303-7

Second Edition

Typeset in Revival BT and Adobe's The Mix

American Psychiatric Publishing, Inc.
1000 Wilson Boulevard
Arlington, VA 22209-3901
www.appi.org

Contents

Questions

Answer Guide

Page numbers in the Study Guide refer to *The American Psychiatric Publishing Textbook of Neuropsychiatry and Behavioral Neurosciences,* Fifth Edition.
Visit **www.appi.org** for more information about this textbook.

CHAPTER 1

Cellular and Molecular Biology of the Neuron

Select the single best response for each question.

1.1 Glial cells are divided into three classes (astrocytes, oligodendrocytes, and microglia) with various different neurophysiological functions. All of the following are functions of astrocytes *except*

A. Structural "scaffolding" of the brain.
B. Formation of the blood-brain barrier.
C. Guidance of neuronal migration during brain development.
D. Cell-cell signaling, often over long distances.
E. Production of the myelin sheath.

1.2 Which of the following statements regarding the electrochemical events involved in the generation of action potentials is *false*?

A. Na^+ and Cl^- are strongly concentrated outside the neuronal cell membrane.
B. K^+ is strongly concentrated within the neuronal cell membrane.
C. At rest, voltage-gated K^+ and Cl^- channels remain closed to preserve equilibrium.
D. The baseline membrane potential is between –50 and –75 mV.
E. Depolarization is only approximately a millisecond because of time-dependent inactivation of Na^+ channels.

1.3 Which of the following statements regarding the neurophysiology of signaling between neurons is *true*?

A. Chemical synapses are formed by gap junctions.
B. Most central nervous system (CNS) synaptic connections are mediated by electrical synapses.
C. Glial cells are connected by gap junctions.
D. Chemical synapses are limited in that they do not allow for signal modulation.
E. Chemical synapses are solely excitatory.

1.4 The two major classes of neurotransmitters are small-molecule transmitters (which mediate fast synaptic transmission and are stored in small, clear vesicles) and neuropeptides (which modulate synaptic transmission and are stored in large, dense-core vesicles). All of the following are classified as small-molecule transmitters *except*

A. Opioids.
B. γ-Aminobutyric acid (GABA).
C. Acetylcholine.
D. Serotonin.
E. Dopamine.

1.5 The process of neurotransmitter release involves several sequential steps. Potent neurotoxins, such as botulinum and tetanus toxin, exert their effects by blocking which step in this cascade of events?

A. Vesicle docking in active zones.
B. Priming.
C. Fusion/exocytosis.
D. Endocytosis.
E. Synaptic vesicle refilling.

1.6 The process of neural development begins with proliferative zones, which line the lumen of the developing ventricular system. All of the following statements regarding neuronal development and migration are true *except*

A. The ventricular zone (VZ), adjacent to the ventricular lumen, contains pseudostratified columnar epithelial cells, now called radial glial cells.
B. A second proliferative zone, the subventricular zone (SVZ), appears just above the VZ.
C. VZ precursor cells are the source of SVZ progenitor cells.
D. SVZ cells are bipolar and maintain physical contact with the pial and ventricular surfaces.
E. Radial glial cells can generate neurons before transforming into astrocytes.

1.7 In the development of synapses, there are three classes of signals that regulate synaptic formation: adhesion molecules, diffusible molecules, and molecules secreted from glial cells. Which of the following is considered to be one of the diffusible molecules?

A. Brain-derived neurotrophic factor (BDNF).
B. Integrins.
C. Nectins.
D. Cadherins.
E. Ephrins.

1.8 Apoptosis is a genetically programmed mechanism of cell death that is crucial to brain development. Which of the following is *not* a component of apoptosis?

A. Cytoplasmic shrinkage.
B. Chromatin condensation.
C. Degradation of neuronal DNA.
D. Dependence on RNA and protein synthesis.
E. An active inflammatory response.

1.9 Glutamate-mediated excitotoxicity is an important process affecting many neuropsychiatric illnesses. Which of the following statements regarding this important mechanism is *false*?

A. Excitotoxicity is mediated by Na^+ entry via α-amino-3-hydroxy-5-methylisoxazole-4-propionic acid (AMPA) channels.
B. Excitotoxicity is the probable mechanism in neuronal loss in stroke.
C. Neuronal depolarization evokes increases in glutamate release.
D. Sustained entry of Ca^{2+} into cells through AMPA channels results in delayed excitotoxicity.
E. Injured neurons show excess levels of intracellular Ca^{2+}.

CHAPTER 2

Functional Neuroanatomy: Neuropsychological Correlates of Cortical and Subcortical Damage

Select the single best response for each question.

2.1 The left and right hemispheres of the human brain differ in several fundamental ways. All of the following statements concerning lateral specialization are true *except*

A. In the vast majority of people, the left hemisphere is specialized for language and for processing verbally coded information.
B. The right hemisphere processes nonverbal information such as visual patterns or auditory signals.
C. The left hemisphere is specialized for the perception of our bodies in space.
D. The right hemisphere is dedicated to the mapping of feeling states.
E. The left hemisphere is involved in the processing of verbal information apprehended through either auditory or visual channels.

2.2 There are several major subdivisions of the temporal lobe. Where is the hippocampus located?

A. Nonmesial portion of the temporal lobe.
B. The mesial temporal lobe.
C. Posterior portion of the superior temporal gyrus.
D. Temporal pole.
E. Inferotemporal region.

2.3 With respect to the nature of amnesia associated with hippocampal damage, all of the following statements are true *except*

A. Neuropsychological findings have demonstrated selective impairments in relational memory.
B. The hippocampal system mediates long-term relational memory.
C. There is a consistent relationship between the side of the hippocampal lesion and the type of learning impairment.
D. The hippocampal system plays a role in the learning of perceptuomotor skills.
E. The hippocampal system is not the principal repository for old memories.

2.4 The amygdala plays an important role in

A. The recognition of emotion.
B. The classical conditioning of autonomic responses.
C. The processing of stimuli that communicate emotional significance in social situations.
D. The decision-making process.
E. All of the above.

2.5 Optic ataxia…

A. Is a disturbance of visually guided reaching behavior.
B. Is a deficit of visual scanning.
C. Consists of an inability to direct the gaze voluntarily toward a stimulus located in the peripheral vision to bring it into central vision.
D. Is necessary for the development of visual disorientation.
E. Is characterized by patients having difficulty pointing to sound sources.

2.6 Which of the following statements concerning Wernicke's aphasia is *false*?

A. It is hallmarked by fluent, paraphasic speech.
B. Patients exhibit impaired repetition.
C. Patients' aural comprehension remains intact.
D. Patients produce speech without hesitation.
E. The phrase length and melodic contour of utterances are normal.

2.7 Which of the following statements concerning Broca's aphasia is *true*?

A. Patients have fluent speech.
B. The aphasia is characterized by long utterances.
C. There is a marked increase in the density of words per unit time.
D. Paraphasias are uncommon.
E. A defect in repetition is invariably present.

2.8 The dorsolateral prefrontal cortex region of the brain…

A. Occupies Brodmann areas 11, 12, 25, and 32.
B. Is involved in working memory.
C. Mediates long-term storage of information.
D. May be assessed for deficits by asking the patient important historical dates in his or her life (e.g., date of birth, wedding anniversary, birthdates of children).
E. None of the above.

2.9 The basal ganglia are a set of deep gray nuclear structures which include which of the following?

A. Lenticular nucleus.
B. Putamen.
C. Caudate nucleus.
D. Globus pallidus.
E. All of the above.

CHAPTER 3

Nervous, Endocrine, and Immune System Interactions in Psychiatry

Select the single best response for each question.

3.1 A major branch point in classification of immune system cells is the distinction between "lymphoid" and "myeloid" cell lines. Which of the following cell types is classified as lymphoid?

A. B cells.
B. Monocytes.
C. Neutrophils.
D. Basophils.
E. Eosinophils.

3.2 Cytokines are immune signaling factors which serve as important mediators in immunity and disease. Many of the cytokines have important relationships to psychiatric symptoms and illnesses. Which of the cytokines is produced by macrophages, fibroblasts, lymphoblastoid cells, and virally infected cells and includes in its activities the increased expression of histocompatibility molecules, induction of viral resistance, and stimulation of natural killer cells?

A. Interleukin 1.
B. Interleukin 2.
C. Interleukin 6.
D. Interferon α.
E. Interferon β.

3.3 The distinction between innate (or natural) immunity and acquired immunity is based on the necessity for prior exposure to the antigen. These two complementary systems are mediated by several soluble mediators. Which of the following soluble mediators is associated with innate immunity?

A. Interferon γ.
B. Interleukin 1 (IL-1).
C. Interleukin 2 (IL-2).
D. Interleukin 4 (IL-4).
E. Interleukin 10 (IL-10).

3.4 Acquired immunity is a complex process that follows exposure to an antigen, so that the antigen is "remembered" by the immune system. All of the following are phases in the mechanism of the acquired immune response *except*

A. Induction phase.
B. Activation phase.
C. Effector phase.
D. Memory phase.
E. Complement protein amplification phase.

3.5 The organism's immunological response to stress is conceptualized in both acute and chronic time frames, with some differences in immunological mediator function in these two responses. Although this work is based on animal models, the immunological response to stress may have important correlates in psychiatric illness. Which of the following changes is characteristic of *chronic* stress in laboratory animals?

A. Decreased antibody production.
B. Decreased phagocyte function.
C. Increased acute phase proteins.
D. Activation of nuclear factor–kappa B (NFkB).
E. Increased number of circulating natural killer (NK) cells.

3.6 In human studies, the differentiation of acute vs. chronic stress response reveals some differences in immune functions but also some similarities. Which of the following is associated with chronic stress but not acute stress in human subjects?

A. Decreased natural killer (NK) cell activity.
B. Increased production of proinflammatory cytokines.
C. Increased white blood cell count.
D. Increased antibody titer to viruses.
E. Decreased antibody response to vaccine.

3.7 Rheumatoid arthritis (RA) is a systemic illness with much psychiatric comorbidity in clinical practice. Which of the following statements regarding the immunological aspects of RA is *true*?

A. Rheumatoid factor (RF) positive patients show a strong association between stressful events and disease onset.
B. RA patients typically demonstrate profound increases in cortisol following surgery and other major interventions.
C. Treatment of depression in RA is associated with improved mood but no improvement in pain or physical disability.
D. In RA, both joint swelling and depression are associated with increased levels of the soluble interleukin-2 receptor (sIL-2R).
E. RA is associated with an excess of T helper 1 (Th1) cell activation.

3.8 A reported syndrome of "sickness behavior" or "neurovegetative syndrome" may be seen with the therapeutic use of cytokines that overlaps with major depression phenomenologically. There is also a "mood/cognitive" syndrome seen in these patients. This may lead to clinical ambiguity in the management of complex clinical conditions; e.g., the treatment of depression in a patient with hepatitis C who is also receiving the cytokine interferon-α. Which of the following statements regarding behavioral symptoms in interferon therapy is *true*?

A. The "mood/cognitive" syndrome occurs early in interferon-α therapy and is nonresponsive to antidepressants.
B. The "neurovegetative syndrome" usually occurs early in interferon treatment and is responsive to antidepressants.
C. The "mood/cognitive" syndrome is associated with suppression of corticotropin-releasing hormone (CRH) pathways.
D. The "mood/cognitive" syndrome is associated with normal serotonin metabolism and altered dopamine metabolism.
E. The "mood/cognitive" syndrome appears late in interferon treatment and is responsive to antidepressants.

CHAPTER 4

Bedside Neuropsychiatry: Eliciting the Clinical Phenomena of Neuropsychiatric Illness

Select the single best response for each question.

4.1 Some physical anomalies are stable through childhood and give clues to abnormal neurodevelopment in adulthood. A scale that is in common use to note these anomalies is called the Waldrop scale. Which of the following minor physical anomalies is *not* included in this scale?

A. Small nails.
B. Wide-spaced eyes.
C. Adherent ear lobes.
D. Furrowed tongue.
E. Abnormal palm crease.

4.2 Palilalia is defined as

A. The patient's repetition of speech of another person.
B. The patient's automatic repetition of his or her own word or phrase.
C. The patient's speech marked by impulsive utterances of stereotyped or simple responses with no aphasic or echolalic features.
D. Loss of the production or recognition of affective elements of speech.
E. A disorder of fluency in which discourse, rather than purely articulation, is disturbed by a range of deficits in speech pragmatics, motor control, and attention.

4.3 Tremors are rhythmic, regular, oscillating movements. In rest tremor, the movement is present distally when the limb is supported and relaxed; action reduces the intensity of the tremor. The most common disorder associated with this tremor is

A. Hereditary, essential tremor.
B. Anxiety.
C. Metabolic encephalopathy.
D. Medication induced (caffeine, lithium).
E. Parkinson's disease.

4.4 If a patient exhibits sudden jerks, sometimes simple, but sometimes as complex as well-organized voluntary movements, that persist in sleep, you would call these movements

A. Chorea.
B. Myoclonus.
C. Asterixis.
D. Tics.
E. Stereotypies.

4.5 In conducting a neurological examination of a patient, the examiner brings the reflex hammer toward the patient's mouth then to the side. What primitive reflex is being assessed?

A. Suck.
B. Rooting.
C. Snout.
D. Avoidance.
E. Nuchocephalic.

4.6 Abulia may be defined as

A. The patient's continuing into present activity the elements of previous actions.
B. The patient's incapacity to carry out a sequential or ordered set of actions toward a unitary goal in the presence of the necessary objects.
C. The patient's lack of will, which in less severe form may include slowness, delayed response, laconic speech, and reduced initiative and effort.
D. The patient's incapacity to sustain activities that he or she was quite capable of beginning.
E. None of the above.

4.7 A recently developed screening test, called the Frontal Assessment Battery, was developed by Dubois et al. (2000) primarily to assess

A. Executive cognitive dysfunction.
B. Dementia.
C. Focal cognitive syndromes.
D. HIV-related dementia.
E. Memory.

CHAPTER 5

Electrodiagnostic Techniques in Neuropsychiatry

Select the single best response for each question.

5.1 The electroencephalography (EEG) frequencies standard in clinical practice are reported in terms of particular ranges with corresponding Greek letters. All of the following ranges and referenced Greek-letter pairs are correct *except*

A. Gamma: >30 Hz.
B. Beta: 12–30 Hz.
C. Alpha: 8–12 Hz.
D. Theta: 4–7 Hz.
E. Delta: <1 Hz.

5.2 Electroencephalography (EEG) has been used to establish electrophysiological correlates in panic disorder; indeed, because of its episodic nature, panic disorder is sometimes formulated as a seizure-like phenomenon. All of the following symptoms are common to simple partial seizures and panic attacks *except*

A. Fear.
B. Bradycardia.
C. Derealization.
D. Diaphoresis.
E. Abdominal discomfort.

5.3 Seizure activity and episodic aggression have been found to be clinically associated. As such, electroencephalography (EEG) may be useful clinically in evaluation of such patients. All of the following statements are true *except*

A. EEG abnormalities have been reported in approximately 50% of patients with antisocial personality disorder.
B. EEG abnormalities are more common in nonhabitual aggressors vs. habitual aggressors.
C. Bilateral paroxysmal EEG features are common in subjects who attack strangers.
D. An abnormal EEG may predict a favorable response to anticonvulsants in violent subjects.
E. Anticonvulsants may be beneficial in violent subjects even if the EEG is normal.

5.4 Electroencephalography (EEG) may be of use in the evaluation of cognitive disorders. Which of the following statements regarding the EEG in this group of illnesses is *true*?

A. A drop in background alpha of 1–2 Hz over a short period of time is not indicative of delirium as long as the alpha rhythm remains in the normal range.
B. Low-voltage beta activity increases in adults up to age 60 years and remains stable thereafter.
C. Mild diffuse slowing is pathological in individuals older than 75 years.
D. Focal delta activity in the anterior temporal areas is rare in patients older than 60 years.
E. EEG slowing is correlated with the severity of dementia and the number of senile plaques in Alzheimer's disease.

5.5 Quantitative electroencephalography (QEEG) may have utility in the understanding of neuropsychiatric disorders and may even have prognostic significance. All of the following statements are true *except*

A. Schizophrenic patients have more delta activity compared with control subjects.
B. Delta activity is more pronounced in schizophrenic patients treated with antipsychotics.
C. Increased delta activity is present in children with high genetic loading for schizophrenia.
D. Alpha and beta power during photic stimulation is decreased in patients with presenile dementia.
E. Intoxication, delirium, and dementia are associated with increased delta activity.

5.6 Mild head injury is an oft-encountered problem in neuropsychiatric practice. Electroencephalography (EEG) may be helpful in evaluating these cases. Which of the following is *not* true of the EEG in head injury?

A. EEG has been shown to correlate with the admission Glasgow Coma Scale score for head injury.
B. Head injury features reduced theta activity.
C. Head injury features reduced beta activity.
D. Head injury features reduced alpha activity.
E. Frontal and temporal EEG abnormalities are common in mild head injury.

5.7 Pharmaco-electroencephalography (pharmaco-EEG) in clinical applications offers an attractive technique to fine-tune drug development, and is likely to play an expanded role in the future of applied psychopharmacology. All of the following statements are true *except*

A. Decreased quantitative electroencephalography (QEEG) theta and alpha activity have been reported in schizophrenic patients treated with high-potency antipsychotics.
B. Slow alpha changes identify nonresponders vs. responders to antipsychotics.
C. Medication-associated increases in beta waves correlate with decrease in depression symptoms.
D. QEEG profile after a single dose of an acetylcholinesterase inhibitor predicted cognitive modifications in dementia patients.
E. With antipsychotic treatment, increased QEEG alpha activity correlates with a favorable clinical response.

5.8 Evoked potentials, particularly the P300 potential, may be useful in the diagnosis and management of neuropsychiatric illness. All of the following statements are true *except*

A. The most consistent P300 finding in schizophrenia is a reduction in amplitude.
B. In schizophrenia, P300 abnormalities are present in nonmedicated and medicated patients.
C. P300 abnormalities correlate with the amount of negative symptoms and formal thought disorder in schizophrenia.
D. In schizophrenia, asymmetrical auditory P300 reduction is frequently reported, with smaller amplitudes over the right temporal region.
E. P300 abnormalities have been reported in relatives of schizophrenia patients and high-risk subjects for psychosis.

CHAPTER 6

The Neuropsychological Evaluation

Select the single best response for each question.

6.1 Depressed patients without psychotic features often underperform, in comparison with control subjects, in all of the following functional areas *except*

A. Measures of speed of processing.
B. Mental flexibility.
C. Executive function.
D. Memory.
E. None of the above.

6.2 One approach to neuropsychological testing is the use of a fixed battery of tests. Which of the following is an advantage of such an approach?

A. It allows the neuropsychologist to focus on a specific area of difficulty.
B. It enables the examiner to cover an area relevant for a diagnosis.
C. The patient receives a broad-based examination.
D. The examination usually will be brief, lasting only 1–2 hours.
E. All aspects of neuropsychological functioning will be examined.

6.3 Patients may usually be grouped into one of the standard aphasia syndromes. Which of the following is *not* one of these syndromes?

A. Spontaneous aphasia.
B. Receptive aphasia.
C. Expressive aphasia.
D. Conduction aphasia.
E. Anomic aphasia.

6.4 Memory is a cognitive function frequently impaired by brain disorders. Which of the following statements regarding the neuropsychological effects of brain injury is *true*?

A. Left-hemispheric lesions are most likely to produce visuospatial memory impairments.
B. In most cases of brain injury, patients with memory impairment usually perform poorly on tests of fund of information or recall of remote events.
C. Most brain-injured patients will retain information learned before the injury as compared with new learning.
D. Right-hemispheric lesions are most likely to produce primarily verbal memory deficits.
E. Patients frequently will have anterograde amnesia without significant retrograde amnesia.

6.5 Executive functions include the ability to formulate a goal, to plan, to carry out goal-directed plans effectively, and to monitor and self-correct spontaneously and reliably. All of the following tests measure aspects of executive functioning *except*

A. The Tower of London.
B. Behavioral Assessment of the Dysexecutive Syndrome (BADS).
C. Twenty Questions test.
D. The Wisconsin Card Sorting Test (WCST).
E. The Complex Figure test.

6.6 Which of the following tests is a self-report of symptoms associated with psychiatric disorders when they occur at high frequency levels?

A. The Hiscock and Hiscock Digit Memory Test.
B. The Symptom Checklist–90—Revised (SCL-90-R).
C. The Test of Memory Malingering (TOMM).
D. The Symptom Validity Test.
E. The Tinkertoy Test.

CHAPTER 7

Clinical and Functional Imaging in Neuropsychiatry

Select the single best response for each question.

7.1 Neuroimaging has revolutionized the clinical practice of neuropsychiatry. For many psychiatric conditions, information obtained from brain imaging studies may assist with differential diagnosis, suggest a treatment plan, and inform prognosis. Which of the following conditions would *not* be considered an indication for neuroimaging?

A. Poison/toxin exposure.
B. Traumatic brain injury.
C. Dementia.
D. Catatonia.
E. Relapse of established psychotic illness.

7.2 Noncontrast computed tomography (CT) of the brain remains the standard neuroimaging in neuropsychiatric practice for many conditions. Which of the following tissue types has a characteristic white appearance in noncontrast CT scans?

A. Water.
B. Cerebrospinal fluid.
C. Gray matter.
D. Clotted blood.
E. White matter.

7.3 In magnetic resonance imaging (MRI), spin echo pulse sequences include T1-weighted, T2-weighted, and fluid-attenuated inversion recovery (FLAIR) sequences. Generally, the T2 and FLAIR sequences are superior for the interpretation of neuropathology. Which of the following tissues appears differently in T2-weighted vs. FLAIR images?

A. Cerebrospinal fluid.
B. Bone.
C. Gray matter.
D. White matter.
E. Blood.

7.4 The neuropsychiatrist must frequently choose the most clinically appropriate neuroimaging modality for the case at hand. Which of the following clinical conditions is preferentially imaged with computed tomography (CT), as opposed to magnetic resonance imaging (MRI)?

A. Subcortical lesions.
B. Poison/toxin exposure.
C. Acute hemorrhage.
D. Eating disorders.
E. Demyelinating disease.

7.5 Positron emission tomography (PET) and single-photon emission computed tomography (SPECT) offer a more dynamic assessment of neuropsychiatric illnesses because of their sensitivity to neural function, not just anatomical structure. Which of the following neuronal functions can be assessed with PET but not with SPECT?

A. Glucose uptake (regional cerebral metabolic rate [rCMR]).
B. Blood flow (regional cerebral blood flow [rCBF]).
C. Serotonin transporter binding.
D. Serotonin receptor binding.
E. Acetylcholine nicotinic receptor binding.

7.6 In the clinical application of positron emission tomography (PET) and single-photon emission computed tomography (SPECT), technical and logistical considerations may make one method preferable to the other. Which of the following statements is *false*?

A. PET has higher spatial resolution than SPECT.
B. PET nearly eliminates attenuation artifacts.
C. SPECT is more widely available and less expensive than PET.
D. Reimbursement for PET is limited to its use for differentiating between Alzheimer's disease and Lewy body dementia.
E. On-site cyclotrons are no longer typically needed for PET scanners.

7.7 One of the most useful applications of functional imaging is in the evaluation of dementia, where functional imaging may assist in elucidating the type of dementia to guide early treatment. All of the following statements are true *except*

A. Alzheimer's disease features bilateral posterior temporoparietal decreased perfusion/metabolism.
B. With progression of Alzheimer's disease, frontal lobes also exhibit decreased perfusion/metabolism.
C. In Alzheimer's disease, occipital cortex is usually preserved.
D. Positron emission tomography (PET)/single-photon emission computed tomography (SPECT) of Parkinson's dementia can be clearly distinguished from SPECT/PET of Alzheimer's disease.
E. SPECT/PET can readily differentiate Alzheimer's disease from frontotemporal dementia (FTD).

7.8 Regarding the use of single-photon emission computed tomography (SPECT)/positron emission tomography (PET) studies in vascular disease, which of the following statements is *true*?

A. Small vessel disease (e.g., Binswanger's disease) has a highly specific SPECT/PET appearance.
B. In acute stroke, SPECT is preferred to CT, because CT is insufficiently accurate in identifying hemorrhagic stroke.
C. Compromised vascular reserve, which may be normal on baseline SPECT, may be visualized following intravenous injection of acetazolamide.
D. Arterioles distal to an obstruction dilate robustly following intravenous injection of acetazolamide.
E. Multi-infarct dementia features multiple moderate-sized defects with diffuse boundaries.

CHAPTER 8

Epidemiological and Genetic Aspects of Neuropsychiatric Disorders

Select the single best response for each question.

8.1 The probability that an individual will develop a disease over a specified time is known as

A. Prevalence.
B. Incidence.
C. Rate.
D. Risk.
E. None of the above.

8.2 A number of research strategies have been developed to elucidate genetic and epidemiological aspects of neuropsychiatric disorders. Which of the following is used to determine the genetic contribution to a disorder?

A. Family studies.
B. Twin studies.
C. High-risk studies.
D. Segregation analysis.
E. Linkage analysis.

8.3 Which of the following statements concerning single-nucleotide polymorphisms (SNPs) is *false*?

A. SNPs are DNA sequence variations.
B. SNPs occur when a single nucleotide (A, T, C, or G) in the genome sequence is altered.
C. SNPs can be in noncoding regions.
D. SNPs can be in genes that affect disease susceptibility.
E. SNPs result from a mutation in a restriction enzyme site.

8.4 All of the following statements concerning the genetics of Huntington's disease (HD) are true *except*

A. It is transmitted in an autosomal dominant fashion.
B. The gene responsible for HD was mapped to the short arm of chromosome 4.
C. Heterozygous inactivation of the HD gene as a result of chromosomal translocation is associated with an abnormal phenotype.
D. The genetic abnormality responsible for HD was identified as a CAG trinucleotide-repeat expansion in the first exon of a novel gene.
E. Age at onset of HD was found to be inversely related to the length of trinucleotide repeats in the gene.

8.5 Which of the following statements about epidemiological findings in Parkinson's disease (PD) is *true?*

A. PD affects about 1% of adults older than 60 years.
B. The prevalence estimate of PD is 900 in 100,000.
C. The average age at onset of PD is 70 years but may be decreasing.
D. PD affects men and women equally.
E. Early-onset PD accounts for 2%–3% of patients.

8.6 Epidemiological findings concerning autism include all of the following *except*

A. Onset typically occurs before age 3 years.
B. The overall rate of autism in second-degree relatives of children with autism is 0.2%.
C. The male-to-female ratio is 1.5 to 1.0.
D. Rates of autism in siblings of affected individuals are in the range of 2%–6%.
E. The concordance rate for monozygotic twins has been estimated to be between 36% and 91%.

8.7 Which of the following factors is associated with a lower risk of developing Alzheimer's disease (AD)?

A. Traumatic brain injury (TBI).
B. Chronic inflammation.
C. Female sex.
D. Cigarette smoking.
E. Higher educational level.

8.8 Family studies of bipolar disorder have demonstrated all of the following findings *except*

A. A sevenfold increase in lifetime risk for bipolar disorder in families with the disorder compared with family members of control subjects.
B. Recurrence risks were found to be higher in females, either of the relative or of the bipolar proband.
C. The age at onset of the first manic or depressive episode has been shown to be earlier in the younger generation of two generations of affected relative pairs.
D. The risk for bipolar disorder appears to be especially elevated in the relatives of probands with early-onset disorder.
E. The risk for bipolar disorder increases with the number of psychiatrically ill relatives.

8.9 High-risk studies of obsessive-compulsive disorder (OCD) in children and adolescents have revealed which of the following?

A. Children with Sydenham's chorea show higher rates of OCD symptoms.
B. Females with early-onset OCD have persistent and severe symptoms.
C. Females with early-onset OCD have a higher incidence of birth complications than males.
D. Early-onset OCD predicts a lower rate of Tourette's disorder and tics in relatives.
E. After exclusion of Tourette's disorder from OCD probands, tics are not found to be more prevalent in OCD families.

8.10 A 22-year-old female patient whom you are treating is concerned that she may develop schizophrenia, given that her mother has been treated for many years for paranoid schizophrenia. She asks you about her risk for developing the illness. The patient is an only child, and her biological father has no psychiatric history. This patient's risk rate is

A. 6%.
B. 13%.
C. 25%.
D. 46%.
E. 53%.

CHAPTER 9

Neuropsychiatric Aspects of Pain Management

Select the single best response for each question.

9.1 Pain is processed by a series of neural tissues that are classified as providing ascending modulation, central processing, or descending inhibition. Which of the following structures is *not* involved in central processing?

A. Spinothalamic tracts.
B. Anterior cingulate gyrus.
C. Insular cortex.
D. Prefrontal cortex.
E. Somatosensory cortex.

9.2 Within central processing, the "medial" system is responsible for generating the affective/emotional component of pain, while the "lateral" system is responsible for the discriminative sensory components. Which of the following structures is part of the medial system?

A. Primary somatosensory cortex (SI).
B. Secondary somatosensory cortex (SII).
C. Anterior cingulate.
D. Parietal cortex.
E. Premotor cortex.

9.3 The relationship between pain and mood disorders is of great clinical relevance to neuropsychiatrists, who frequently treat patients with these comorbid conditions. All of the following statements are true *except*

A. Patients with pain score higher on measures of depression than do patients without pain.
B. In cancer patients, depressive symptoms are more highly correlated with pain than with a history of previous clinical depression.
C. Depression is the most common psychiatric diagnosis among chronic pain patients.
D. The presence or absence of mood symptoms has a differential effect on the opioid responsiveness of pain.
E. Emotional aspects of pain, such as depression, are modulated by the insular cortex.

9.4 Many chemicals present in blood and tissue are algesic. Which of the following substances does *not* itself directly excite primary noxious afferents?

A. Prostaglandins.
B. Serotonin.
C. Histamine.
D. Acetylcholine.
E. Bradykinin.

9.5 The dorsal horn of the spinal cord is divided into different laminae, each with specific roles in neural transmission. Which of these laminae is also known as the substantia gelatinosa and is the site of spinal cord opiate analgesia?

A. Lamina I.
B. Lamina II.
C. Lamina III.
D. Lamina IV.
E. Lamina X.

9.6 Which of the following laminae does not contribute axons to the spinothalamic tract?

A. Lamina I.
B. Lamina IV.
C. Lamina V.
D. Lamina VII.
E. Lamina X.

9.7 Which of the following analgesics is not a cyclooxygenase inhibitor?

A. Acetaminophen.
B. Aspirin.
C. Indomethacin.
D. Diclofenac.
E. Keterolac.

9.8 Treatment of pain states may be an appropriate application of tricyclic antidepressants (TCAs). Unfortunately, a host of cardiac concerns make electrocardiogram (ECG) monitoring necessary with these agents. Which of the following is *not* a characteristic ECG change associated with TCAs?

A. Flattened T-wave.
B. Prolonged Q-T interval.
C. Prolonged QRS interval.
D. Prolonged PR interval.
E. Elevated S-T segment.

9.9 Anticonvulsants are an often helpful class of medications for neuropathic pain. Unfortunately, they are well known to be associated with a series of side effects that may limit their use. Which of the following agents is associated with cognitive slowing and renal stones?

A. Topiramate.
B. Carbamazepine.
C. Levetiracetam.
D. Gabapentin.
E. Lamotrigine.

CHAPTER 10

Neuropsychiatric Aspects of Disorders of Attention

Select the single best response for each question.

10.1 "An alert state in which individuals are aware of self and environment" is a definition of

A. Attentional capacity.
B. Consciousness.
C. Selective attention.
D. Response selection and executive control.
E. Sustained attention.

10.2 A number of different brain regions are involved in attentional processes. Which brain region plays a pivotal role in attention by contributing important energetic components of drive and motivation?

A. Dorsolateral prefrontal cortex.
B. Reticular activating system (RAS).
C. Hypothalamus.
D. Anterior cingulate gyrus.
E. Orbitomedial prefrontal circuit.

10.3 A number of tasks place demands on attentional capacity and focus because of the requirement to divide attention or to inhibit interfering stimuli or responses. An example is a test in which the subject is required to name the color of a word while ignoring the actual word. What is the name of this test?

A. Wisconsin Card Sorting Test.
B. Trail Making Test.
C. Controlled Word Association Test.
D. Continuous Performance Test.
E. Stroop Test.

10.4 A number of psychophysiological and neuroimaging techniques have been used to assess the neurobiological substrates of attention. A test that measures the random thermal motion of water in brain tissue has been used to examine brain dysfunction in a clinical population. What is this test called?

A. Event-related potential (ERP).
B. Functional magnetic resonance imaging (fMRI).
C. Diffusion tensor imaging (DTI).
D. Electroencephalogram (EEG).
E. Autonomic studies.

10.5 Neglect and deficits in attention are important clinical findings in patients with neuropsychiatric disorders. Which of the following statements concerning these impairments is *false*?

A. Neglect usually occurs relative to the right side of space, which illustrates the importance of the dominant hemisphere in spatial attention.
B. Hemi-inattention and neglect are manifestations of unilateral brain lesions.
C. Lesions affecting the reticular system that produce neglect also involve significant arousal and activation impairments.
D. Unilateral basal ganglia damage often results in impairments of both hemi-attention and intention.
E. Cingulate lesions are more likely to affect intention than sensory selective attention.

10.6 Which of the following statements concerning attention-deficit/hyperactivity disorder (ADHD) is *false*?

A. For the most part, patients with ADHD have normal intelligence.
B. In ADHD, the attention deficit results from susceptibility to distraction.
C. Impaired sustained attention is a primary feature of ADHD.
D. Children with ADHD exhibit more errors of both omission and commission on the Continuous Performance Test than do children without ADHD.
E. Patients with ADHD do not exhibit major cognitive dysfunction.

C H A P T E R 1 1

Neuropsychiatric Aspects of Delirium

Select the single best response for each question.

11.1 The diagnostic criteria for delirium as reflected in the DSM series have evolved significantly over time. Which version first specifically included dysexecutive symptoms in the criteria for delirium?

A. DSM-I (American Psychiatric Association 1952).
B. DSM-II (American Psychiatric Association 1968).
C. DSM-III-R (American Psychiatric Association 1987).
D. DSM-IV (American Psychiatric Association 1994).
E. None of the above.

11.2 Misdiagnosis of delirium, a common clinical problem, has been found to be more likely among certain patient populations. Which of the following clinical attributes is *not* a risk factor for such misdiagnosis?

A. Hyperactive patient presentation.
B. Advanced patient age.
C. Sensory impairments.
D. Preexisting dementia.
E. Intensive care setting.

11.3 The distinction between delirium and dementia is rendered problematic by several overlapping symptoms that are common to these two cognitive disorders. Which dementia syndrome, characterized by fluctuating symptom severity, visual hallucinations, attentional impairment, altered state of consciousness, and delusions, is particularly difficult to distinguish from delirium?

A. Dementia due to hypothyroidism.
B. Dementia due to HIV disease.
C. Alzheimer's dementia.
D. Vascular dementia.
E. Lewy body dementia.

11.4 In their study examining differences in symptom profile between patients with delirium and patients with dementia, which of the following symptoms were found by Trzepacz et al. (2002) to be more common in delirium than in dementia?

A. Delusions.
B. Affective lability.
C. Thought process abnormalities.
D. Disorders of short-term memory.
E. Disorders of long-term memory.

11.5 Delirium following stroke is unfortunately a common clinical scenario for the neuropsychiatrist. Which of the following statements regarding the relationship between delirium and stroke is *false?*

A. Delirium complicates the course of acute stroke in nearly 50% of patients.
B. Delirium more commonly follows ischemic than hemorrhagic stroke.
C. Anticholinergic medications carry a particularly high risk of delirium in stroke patients.
D. Poststroke delirium is more common with hemispheric stroke than with brain stem stroke.
E. Delirium is more common following intracerebral rather than subarachnoid hemorrhage or infarct.

11.6 The distinction between "core" and "associated" delirium symptoms may be helpful in understanding delirium phenomenology. Which of the following is considered a "core" symptom of delirium?

A. Illusions.
B. Hallucinations.
C. Delusions.
D. Affective changes.
E. Language disturbances.

11.7 Which of the following atypical antipsychotics, by virtue of its multiple receptor effects (including sedation, anticholinergic properties, and lowering of the seizure threshold), should not be used in delirium?

A. Risperidone.
B. Ziprasidone.
C. Aripiprazole.
D. Clozapine.
E. Olanzapine.

11.8 A final common neural pathway for delirium would encompass both neuroanatomical and neurochemical dimensions. The preponderance of evidence in the literature supports which of the following as the likely final common neural pathway in delirium?

A. Low cholinergic/high dopaminergic state.
B. High cholinergic/high dopaminergic state.
C. High γ-aminobutyric acid (GABA)/low dopaminergic state.
D. Low GABA/high dopaminergic state.
E. Low serotonin/high GABA state.

11.9 Electroencephalography (EEG) may be a helpful diagnostic tool in clarifying cases of delirium, particularly in regard to differential causes of delirium. An EEG pattern of "low-voltage fast activity" is consistent with which of the following delirium etiologies?

A. Anticholinergic toxicity.
B. Post–traumatic brain injury (TBI).
C. Hepatic encephalopathy.
D. Alcohol withdrawal.
E. Hypoxia.

11.10 Delirium rating scales are useful in the diagnosis and monitoring of delirium symptoms. Which of the following statements about the Memorial Delirium Assessment Scale (MDAS) is *false*?

A. It is a severity rating scale designed to be used after a delirium diagnosis has been made.
B. It allows for repeated ratings.
C. Items on the MDAS specifically address temporal onset and symptom fluctuation.
D. The MDAS correlates highly with the Delirium Rating Scale.
E. It has been found useful in distinguishing delirium from other psychiatric illnesses in elderly patients.

C H A P T E R 1 2

Neuropsychiatric Aspects of Aphasia and Related Disorders

Select the single best response for each question.

12.1 The current classification of aphasia syndromes is based on the Wernicke-Geschwind model, which posits that aphasia involves six major language areas. Which of the following is *not* one of the language areas addressed in this model?

A. Fluency.
B. Spelling.
C. Naming.
D. Repetition.
E. Reading.

12.2 In which of the following aphasia syndromes is auditory comprehension abnormal?

A. Anomia.
B. Broca's.
C. Conduction.
D. Transcortical motor.
E. Wernicke's.

12.3 In Broca's aphasia, which of the following language areas is relatively normal?

A. Auditory comprehension.
B. Fluency.
C. Naming.
D. Repetition.
E. Writing comprehension.

12.4 Patients with delirium typically exhibit abnormalities in all of the following language functions *except*

A. Writing.
B. Word-list generation.
C. Motor speech.
D. Automatic speech.
E. Content of speech.

12.5 Which of the following language areas is relatively normal in transcortical motor aphasia but abnormal in Broca's aphasia?

A. Fluency.
B. Naming.
C. Repetition.
D. Writing comprehension.
E. Reading.

12.6 Nonfluent (anterior) aphasia and fluent (posterior) aphasia each are accompanied by a distinct, long-term behavioral syndrome. In anterior aphasia behavioral syndrome, the most common psychiatric symptom is

A. Agitation.
B. Depression.
C. Paranoia.
D. Suicide.
E. Impulsive behavior.

CHAPTER 13

Neuropsychiatric Aspects of Aggression and Impulse-Control Disorders

Select the single best response for each question.

13.1 Which of the following statements regarding violence in the United States is *false*?

A. Homicide is the second leading cause of death among persons 15–24 years of age.
B. Half of all homicides are committed by perpetrators younger than 25 years.
C. The rate of homicide death for men is three times that for women.
D. In domestic violence, men are more likely than women to attack a spouse.
E. In 90% of homicides, perpetrator and victim are of the same race.

13.2 Which of the following is the interview instrument most commonly used to evaluate aggression?

A. Buss-Durkee Hostility Inventory.
B. Hostility and Direction of Hostility Questionnaire.
C. Spielberger State-Trait Anger Expression Inventory.
D. Barratt Impulsiveness Scale.
E. Brown-Goodwin Assessment.

13.3 The hypothalamus has been the focus of much research on the neurobiology of aggression. Which of the following statements is *true*?

A. Stimulation of the anterior hypothalamus in cats produces submissive behavior.
B. Stimulation of the dorsomedial hypothalamus in the cat causes increased predatory attacks on small animals.
C. Lesioning of the ventromedial nucleus in cats results in permanent aggression.
D. Stimulation of the posterior lateral aspect of the hypothalamus in cats prolongs latency of attack.
E. Stimulation of the medial ventral area of the hypothalamus shortens latency of attack.

13.4 In primates, bilateral temporal lobectomy produces the Klüver-Bucy syndrome, which is characterized by all of the following behaviors *except*

A. Hyperorality.
B. Hyposexuality.
C. Absence of fear response.
D. Increased touching.
E. Visual agnosia.

13.5 Which of the following statements regarding serotonin and impulsive aggression is *true*?

A. There is a positive relationship between violent lethal suicidal behavior and 5-hydroxyindoleacetic acid (5-HIAA) in depressed patients.
B. Homicide offenders with a suicide attempt history have a higher concentration of cerebrospinal fluid (CSF) 5-HIAA compared with those without a history of suicide attempts.
C. Low CSF 5-HIAA is related to aggressive behavior independent of suicidal behavior in patient with Axis I disorders.
D. Increased brain stem levels of serotonin and 5-HIAA are found in suicide victims.
E. Increased platelet serotonin receptor sites are found in aggressive subjects.

13.6 A number of inborn metabolic disorders are associated with aggressive and impulsive behavior. Which of the following inherited illnesses is characterized by increased mucopolysaccharide storage?

A. Sanfilippo's syndrome.
B. Phenylketonuria.
C. Lesch-Nyhan syndrome.
D. Prader-Willi syndrome.
E. Vogt's syndrome.

13.7 Neuropsychological testing has revealed correlations between laterality of cerebral dysfunction and specific clinical profiles. On testing, which of the following clinical subgroups shows predominantly right hemisphere dysfunction?

A. Alcoholic individuals with affective disorders.
B. Violent criminals.
C. Alcoholic individuals with personality disorders.
D. Adolescents with conduct disorders.
E. Prisoners with impulsive behaviors.

13.8 Which of the following personality disorders has been found to be common in arsonists?

A. Narcissistic.
B. Histrionic.
C. Schizoid.
D. Borderline.
E. Avoidant.

13.9 Which of the following selective serotonin reuptake inhibitors (SSRIs) has been most extensively studied for the treatment of impulsivity and aggression in borderline personality disorder?

A. Fluvoxamine.
B. Fluoxetine.
C. Sertraline.
D. Citalopram.
E. Paroxetine.

CHAPTER 14

Neuropsychiatric Aspects of Memory and Amnesia

Select the single best response for each question.

14.1 All of the following statements concerning declarative memory are true *except*

A. It is the type of memory assessed by traditional tests of recall and recognition.
B. It is defined as the conscious recollection of words, scenes, faces, stories, and events.
C. It encompasses the subordinate functions of procedural memory, classical conditioning, simple associative learning, and priming.
D. It is usually subdivided into two components: semantic and episodic memory.
E. Its functioning depends on the integrity of the hippocampus and related structures.

14.2 Working memory…

A. Is a form of nondeclarative memory.
B. Is viewed as a single memory buffer.
C. Is a form of declarative memory.
D. Has the central executive as its most important component.
E. Is similar to what in the past was called *long-term memory.*

14.3 Clinical characteristics commonly observed in amnesic patients include all of the following *except*

A. Anterograde amnesia.
B. Aphasia.
C. Retrograde amnesia.
D. Confabulations.
E. Intact intellectual function.

14.4 Depressed patients are more likely than nondepressed patients to have deficits in which of the following domains?

A. Effortful processing.
B. Automatic processing.
C. Nondeclarative memory.
D. Incidental learning.
E. None of the above.

14.5 All of the following statements concerning declarative memory deficits in patients with schizophrenia are true *except*

A. Deficits are more pronounced in tests of recognition than in tests of recall.
B. Patients usually have little or no deficits in nondeclarative memory tests.
C. Procedural learning is usually intact with few or no deficits.
D. Patients have shallow or inefficient encoding of information.
E. Patients frequently exhibit disorganized or inefficient retrieval strategies.

14.6 Which of the following statements concerning dissociative amnesia is *true*?

A. It is frequently diagnosed, especially among patients with "hysterical" disorders.
B. It usually interferes with social or occupational functioning.
C. It is more common in males.
D. It is more common in the elderly than in adolescents or young adults.
E. It usually is transient.

14.7 All of the following medications may adversely affect memory *except*

A. Benzodiazepines.
B. Heterocyclic antidepressants.
C. Neuroleptics.
D. Atypical antipsychotics.
E. Antiparkinsonian agents.

CHAPTER 15

Neuropsychiatric Aspects of Traumatic Brain Injury

Select the single best response for each question.

15.1 Traumatic brain injury (TBI) is associated with profound perturbations of neurotransmitters. Which of the following statements regarding post-TBI neurotransmitter changes is *false*?

A. Excitotoxicity following TBI is mediated by glutamate and acetylcholine.
B. Acute elevations of striatal dopamine post-TBI predict poor functional recovery.
C. Decreased levels of 5-hydroxyindoleacetic acid (5-HIAA) are found with frontotemporal contusions.
D. Decreased levels of 5-HIAA are found with diffuse contusions.
E. TBI is associated acutely with an increase in cholinergic transmission.

15.2 A traumatic brain injury (TBI) patient with eye opening to speech (but not spontaneously), decorticate motor response, and intelligible but incoherent speech would score ___ on the Glasgow Coma Scale.

A. 8.
B. 9.
C. 10.
D. 11.
E. 12.

15.3 Traumatic brain injury (TBI) affecting the frontal lobe is common. Damage to specific frontal lobe regions is associated with particular behavior symptoms. All of the following symptoms are characteristic of the orbitofrontal syndrome *except*

A. Perseveration.
B. Impulsivity.
C. Disinhibition.
D. Hyperactivity.
E. Mood lability.

15.4 Post–traumatic brain injury (TBI) epilepsy presents a clinical challenge, in that several anticonvulsants are themselves associated with impaired cognitive function. Among the following anticonvulsants used to treat post-TBI epilepsy, which is *least* likely to cause adverse effects on cognition?

A. Phenytoin.
B. Carbamazepine.
C. Topiramate.
D. Lamotrigine.
E. Phenobarbital.

15.5 Post–traumatic brain injury (TBI) aggression often exhibits distinctive behavioral features. Which of the following content/context descriptors does *not* characterize the violence committed by these patients?

A. Reactive.
B. Nonreflective.
C. Nonpurposeful.
D. Periodic.
E. Ego-syntonic.

15.6 Clinical guidelines for psychopharmacological treatment of the psychiatric sequelae of traumatic brain injury (TBI) include all of the following *except*

A. Start low (dose) and go slow (with dosage escalations).
B. Continuously reassess clinical status.
C. Monitor for drug–drug interactions.
D. Augment partial responses.
E. Limit doses to less than usual full recommended doses.

15.7 Pathological laughing and/or crying (PLC) is a classic disorder of affective dysregulation that is an infrequent consequence of traumatic brain injury (TBI). Which of the following statements about PLC is *false*?

A. Episodes of crying and/or laughter do not produce a persistent change in mood.
B. Episodes may occur many times a day.
C. Episodes must be provoked by emotionally evocative stimuli.
D. Presentation of symptoms is quite stereotyped.
E. Episodes are uncontrollable.

15.8 Atypical antipsychotics are commonly used in management of the behavioral consequences of traumatic brain injury (TBI). However, the physician must be mindful of adverse drug effects in this vulnerable population. Among the following atypical antipsychotics, which is the *least* likely to produce extrapyramidal side effects (EPS)?

A. Risperidone.
B. Ziprasidone.
C. Quetiapine.
D. Olanzapine.
E. Aripiprazole.

15.9 Which of the following classes of medications is *not* recommended for use in chronically agitated traumatic brain injury (TBI) patients?

A. β-Blockers.
B. Buspirone.
C. Serotonergic antidepressants.
D. Atypical antipsychotics.
E. Benzodiazepines.

CHAPTER 16

Neuropsychiatric Aspects of Seizure Disorders

Select the single best response for each question.

16.1 The International League Against Epilepsy (ILAE) has proposed a five-axis diagnostic scheme to classify seizures. Which of the five axes is used to specify etiology?

A. Axis I.
B. Axis II.
C. Axis III.
D. Axis IV.
E. Axis V.

16.2 In which of the following seizure types is consciousness preserved?

A. Tonic-clonic seizures.
B. Simple partial seizures.
C. Status epilepticus.
D. Absence seizures.
E. Complex partial seizures.

16.3 Which of the following is the major laboratory test used in the diagnostic workup of seizures?

A. Prolactin level.
B. Serum albumin.
C. Serum potassium.
D. Serum calcium.
E. Creatine phosphokinase (CPK).

16.4 Which of the following statements about nonepileptic seizures (pseudoseizures) is *false*?

A. Injury is infrequent.
B. Plantar flexor reflexes are preserved.
C. Postictal features are typical.
D. Sleep-related seizures are infrequent.
E. Restraint accentuates the seizure.

16.5 Which of the following diagnostic clues may help differentiate psychosis due to a central nervous system lesion or seizures from schizophrenic psychosis?

A. Presentation that meets DSM-IV (American Psychiatric Association 1994) criteria.
B. Poor premorbid social history.
C. Gradual change in personality, mood, or ability to function.
D. Rapid fluctuations in mental status.
E. Responsiveness to usual biological or psychological interventions.

16.6 Basic guidelines for treating seizure disorder patients with concomitant psychiatric symptoms include all of the following *except*

A. Preferably use anticonvulsant monotherapy.
B. Start with higher doses of psychotropic medications in order to rapidly treat symptoms.
C. Anticipate possible drug interactions between anticonvulsant and psychotropic medications.
D. Evaluate the need for adjustment of the anticonvulsant.
E. Optimize the addition of psychotropic medication by targeting specific psychiatric symptoms.

C H A P T E R 1 7

Neuropsychiatric Aspects of Sleep and Sleep Disorders

Select the single best response for each question.

17.1 Sleep stages are defined by specific electroencephalographic parameters. Which sleep stage features sleep spindles or K complexes, with high-amplitude delta activity for less than 20% of the epoch?

A. Stage I.
B. Stage II.
C. Stage III.
D. Stage IV.
E. Rapid eye movement (REM).

17.2 Which of the following general statements about sleep architecture is *false*?

A. Sleep is entered through non–rapid eye movement (NREM) sleep.
B. NREM and rapid eye movement (REM) sleep alternate every 90 minutes.
C. Slow-wave sleep dominates the first third of the night.
D. REM sleep dominates the last third of the night.
E. REM episodes are shorter later in the sleep period.

17.3 Sleep disturbances in major depression include all of the following *except*

A. Generalized sleep disturbance.
B. Increase in slow-wave sleep in the first non–rapid eye movement (NREM)–rapid eye movement (REM) cycle.
C. Lengthening of latency to REM sleep.
D. Occurrence of REM sleep earlier in the night.
E. Increase in REM density.

17.4 Although most antidepressants are known to suppress rapid eye movement (REM) sleep, some antidepressants do not have this property. Which of the following antidepressants does not suppress REM sleep?

A. Paroxetine.
B. Fluoxetine.
C. Desipramine.
D. Monoamine oxidase inhibitors.
E. Bupropion.

17.5 Psychophysiological insomnia is a troubling sleep disorder with specific behavioral characteristics. Which of the following is *not* a feature of this condition?

A. Excessive worry about not being able to sleep.
B. Trying too hard to sleep.
C. Rumination.
D. Inability to sleep unless in one's own bed.
E. Increased muscle tension when retiring.

17.6 Disorders of daytime sleepiness can cause great functional impairment and even physically dangerous behavior. Which of the following is the most common cause of excessive daytime sleepiness?

A. Sleep apnea.
B. Narcolepsy.
C. Idiopathic hypersomnia.
D. Kleine-Levin syndrome.
E. Posttraumatic hypersomnia.

17.7 Predisposing factors for obstructive sleep apnea include all of the following *except*

A. Hyperthyroidism and acromegaly.
B. Male sex.
C. Middle age or older.
D. Obesity.
E. Micrognathia or retrognathia.

17.8 Narcolepsy is another sleep disorder associated with great functional impairment. All of the following are features of narcolepsy *except*

A. Excessive daytime sleepiness.
B. Cataplexy.
C. Sleep paralysis.
D. Hypnopompic hallucinations.
E. Hypnagogic hallucinations.

17.9 The parasomnias are a class of behavior disorders occurring during sleep. Which of the following is considered to be the most common parasomnia?

A. Nocturnal seizures.
B. Sleepwalking.
C. Sleep terrors.
D. Nightmares.
E. Bruxism.

17.10 A patient suddenly screams or cries, abruptly sits up in bed, appears to be intensely fearful, is unresponsive to external stimuli, and vocalizes incoherently. Later, the patient is amnestic for the episode. The most likely diagnosis is

A. Nightmare.
B. Rapid eye movement (REM) sleep behavior disorder.
C. Sleepwalking.
D. Rhythmic movement disorder.
E. Sleep terror.

17.11 Rapid eye movement (REM) sleep behavior disorder is a rare condition in which patients "act out their dreams" due to a failure of REM-associated atonia. This condition has been associated with use of all the following medication classes or agents *except*

A. Serotonin antagonists.
B. Tricyclic antidepressants (TCAs).
C. Monoamine oxidase inhibitors (MAOIs).
D. Venlafaxine.
E. Serotonin agonists.

CHAPTER 18

Neuropsychiatric Aspects of Cerebrovascular Disorders

Select the single best response for each question.

18.1 Among the following, which is the least common type of cerebrovascular disease?

A. Ruptured aneurysm.
B. Intracerebral hemorrhage.
C. Lacunae.
D. Cerebral embolism.
E. Atherosclerotic thrombosis.

18.2 The onset of major depression within the first 2 months following a stroke is most common when the stroke affects which of the following brain regions?

A. Right anterior.
B. Right posterior.
C. Left anterior.
D. Left posterior.
E. Bilateral posterior.

18.3 In comparisons of patients with poststroke depression with poststroke patients who did not develop depression, investigators found which of the following to increase the risk of depression following stroke?

A. Older age.
B. Greater subcortical atrophy.
C. Female sex.
D. Lower socioeconomic status.
E. Less education.

18.4 Although poststroke mania occurs much less frequently than does poststroke depression, secondary mania may sometimes develop following a stroke. Poststroke mania is most frequently associated with damage to which of the following brain regions?

A. Left anterior frontal.
B. Left posterior temporal.
C. Left occipital.
D. Bilateral anterior.
E. Right hemisphere.

18.5 Which of the following statements concerning poststroke anxiety disorder is *true*?

A. Few patients with generalized anxiety disorder (GAD) meet criteria for major depression.
B. Late-onset GAD is associated with a history of psychiatric disorder.
C. Depression with anxiety is associated with right cortical lesions.
D. Over time, the strongest correlates of GAD are an absence of social contacts outside the family and dependence on others to perform activities of daily living (ADLs).
E. GAD has not been associated with cortical atrophy.

18.6 Which of the following statements concerning patients with catastrophic reactions to stroke is *false*?

A. Patients have a higher frequency of familial history of psychiatric disorders.
B. Patients have higher rates of major depression.
C. Patients are more likely to be aphasic.
D. Patients more commonly have a personal history of psychiatric disorders.
E. Patients have a higher frequency of basal ganglia lesions.

CHAPTER 19

Neuropsychiatric Aspects of Brain Tumors

Select the single best response for each question.

19.1 The most common type of primary brain tumor is

A. Meningioma.
B. Glioma.
C. Pituitary adenoma.
D. Medulloblastoma.
E. Neurilemmoma.

19.2 The most common primary site for a central nervous system (CNS) metastatic tumor is

A. Lung.
B. Breast.
C. Kidney.
D. Gastrointestinal tract.
E. Skin.

19.3 Tumors of the frontal lobe may be associated with the "dorsolateral prefrontal syndrome." All of the following are features of this syndrome *except*

A. "Pseudopsychopathic" behavior.
B. Apathy.
C. Indifference.
D. Psychomotor retardation.
E. Poor initiation of tasks.

19.4 Although tumors of the temporal lobes may present with symptoms similar to classic schizophrenia, certain phenomenological differences have been noted between the two conditions. Symptoms more typically associated with temporal lobe tumors than with classic schizophrenia include all of the following *except*

A. Visual hallucinations.
B. Olfactory hallucinations.
C. Tactile hallucinations.
D. "Spells" and dreamlike episodes.
E. Flat or inappropriate affect.

19.5 Tumors of the nondominant parietal lobe may produce the constellation of symptoms called Gerstmann's syndrome. Which of the following is *not* a feature of this syndrome?

A. Hemi-neglect.
B. Dysgraphia.
C. Acalculia.
D. Finger agnosia.
E. Left–right confusion.

19.6 Bitemporal hemianopsia, optic atrophy, and diabetes insipidus are symptoms associated with tumors of which region?

A. Pineal.
B. Cerebellum.
C. Basal ganglia.
D. Pituitary.
E. Occipital lobes.

19.7 Systemic findings that should trigger increased suspicion for brain tumor in patients with behavioral symptoms include all of the following *except*

A. Nonfocal neurological signs.
B. Seizures.
C. Headaches.
D. Sensory changes.
E. Nausea and vomiting.

19.8 In treatment of depression in a brain tumor patient who is at risk of seizures, which of the following agents should be avoided?

A. Fluoxetine.
B. Venlafaxine.
C. Maprotiline.
D. Sertraline.
E. Paroxetine.

CHAPTER 20

Neuropsychiatric Aspects of Human Immunodeficiency Virus Infection of the Central Nervous System

Select the single best response for each question.

20.1 Which of the following statements concerning the epidemiology of acquired immunodeficiency syndrome (AIDS) and human immunodeficiency virus (HIV) infection is *false*?

A. In the United States, approximately 950,000 persons are living with HIV.
B. Worldwide, there are 38 million people living with HIV.
C. In the United States, the annual rate of diagnosis of HIV/AIDS has increased approximately 4% over the 2000–2003 time period.
D. Up to 30% of HIV-infected individuals may be expected to develop HIV-1-associated dementia during the course of the infection.
E. In the United States, approximately 930,000 persons have a diagnosis of AIDS.

20.2 The most common opportunistic infection in AIDS, which may present as a focal or diffuse cognitive or affective disturbance, is

A. Syphilis.
B. *Toxoplasma gondii*.
C. Cytomegalovirus.
D. *Cryptococcus neoformans*.
E. Progressive multifocal leukoencephalopathy.

20.3 According to American Academy of Neurology (AAN) criteria for HIV-1-associated minor cognitive/motor disorder, diagnostic cognitive/motor/behavioral dysfunctions include all of the following *except*

A. Impaired attention/concentration.
B. Impaired memory.
C. Slowed movements.
D. Incoordination.
E. Disturbance of consciousness.

20.4 Which of the following statements concerning the treatment of delirium in HIV patients is *true*?

A. In neuroleptic treatment of HIV delirium, initial doses may need to be lower than those used in other medically ill populations.
B. Neuroleptic malignant syndrome is the most common adverse side effect of intravenous haloperidol.
C. Use of intravenous haloperidol to treat delirium is approved by the U.S. Food and Drug Administration.
D. Doses of intravenous medications should not be increased to high levels.
E. Adverse effects of haloperidol in HIV-infected patients are much less frequent if the patient has another coexisting mental disorder due to a general medical condition.

20.5 Which of the following antidepressants should be avoided in treatment of HIV/AIDS depression?

A. Escitalopram.
B. Mirtazapine.
C. Citalopram.
D. Nefazodone.
E. Bupropion.

CHAPTER 21

Neuropsychiatric Aspects of Endocrine Disorders

Select the single best response for each question.

21.1 Cross-sectional and prospective studies have revealed significant cognitive deficits in patients with diabetes mellitus. Which of the following statements concerning diabetes-associated cognitive impairment/decline is *false*?

A. Diabetes increases the risk of both vascular dementia and Alzheimer's disease in older patients.
B. Children with insulin-dependent diabetes mellitus (IDDM) (type I diabetes) suffer from cognitive impairment, with poor metabolic control as a risk factor.
C. Executive function is particularly at risk in IDDM children with disease onset before 4 years of age.
D. Hypoglycemia impairs cognition irreversibly.
E. Greater than 15 years' duration of diabetes increases the risk of cognitive decline.

21.2 The symptoms of hypoglycemia in diabetic patients have significant behavioral components. For classification purposes, these symptoms are divided into the "autonomic" and "neuroglycopenic" symptoms. Which of the following is considered to be an "autonomic" symptom?

A. Confusion.
B. Tremor.
C. Lethargy.
D. Speech changes.
E. Incoordination.

21.3 The metabolic syndrome associated with non-insulin-dependent diabetes mellitus (NIDDM) (type II diabetes) is also seen with the use of atypical antipsychotic agents. All of the following are characteristic of this metabolic syndrome *except*

A. Insulin resistance.
B. Abdominal obesity.
C. Hypertension.
D. Decreased insulin production.
E. Dyslipidemia.

21.4 Treatment of depression in diabetic patients is crucial to promote metabolic stability and to enhance life functioning. All of the following statements are true *except*

A. Remission of depression is achieved in only a small percentage of cases over 5 years.
B. Depression relapses in diabetic patients occur at a rate of one episode per year.
C. Response rates to antidepressant treatment in diabetic patients are only 50% of response rates in nondiabetic patients.
D. Monoamine oxidase inhibitors (MAOIs) exacerbate hypoglycemia and are associated with weight gain.
E. Anticholinergic side effects of some antidepressants can worsen diabetes-related gastroparesis.

21.5 Hypothyroidism is an endocrinological illness of great interest to the neuropsychiatrist and serves as a convenient model for psychiatric symptoms due to systemic illness. Which of the following is the most commonly reported psychiatric symptom in hypothyroidism?

A. Depression.
B. Bipolar disorder.
C. Psychotic disorders.
D. Anxiety disorders.
E. Cognitive disorders.

21.6 Hypothyroidism is classified on a grading scale correlated to clinical and laboratory abnormalities. "Subclinical hypothyroidism," which is associated with depression and is characterized by elevated thyroid-stimulating hormone (TSH), normal levels of thyroid hormones, and an exaggerated TSH response to thyrotropin-releasing hormone (TRH), would be classified as grade ___.

A. I.
B. II.
C. III.
D. IV.
E. V.

21.7 As with hypothyroidism, hyperthyroidism is associated with significant degrees of psychiatric comorbidity. Which of the following is the most common psychiatric manifestation of hyperthyroidism?

A. Psychosis.
B. Cognitive disturbance.
C. Mania.
D. Major depression.
E. Anxiety.

21.8 Corticosteroid-induced psychiatric symptoms are a serious consequence of long-term steroid therapy. Which of the following agents is *not* a recommended pharmacotherapeutic strategy for managing these symptoms?

A. Lamotrigine.
B. Lithium.
C. Tricyclic antidepressants (TCAs).
D. Valproic acid.
E. Olanzapine.

21.9 Hypoparathyroidism is associated with a wide range of psychiatric symptoms. Which of the following psychiatric disorders is the most prevalent in hypoparathyroidism?

A. Mood disorders.
B. Anxiety disorders.
C. Cognitive disorders.
D. Psychotic disorders.
E. Dissociative disorders.

CHAPTER 22

Neuropsychiatric Aspects of Poisons and Toxins

Select the single best response for each question.

22.1 Which of the following solvents produces peripheral neuropathy as its most common adverse side effect?

A. Ethylbenzene.
B. Ethylene glycol.
C. Carbon tetrachloride.
D. Methyl-*n*-butyl ketone.
E. Methanol.

22.2 High plasma aluminum concentrations have been associated with various neuropsychiatric symptoms. Which of the following plasma aluminum levels has been associated with incoordination, intention tremor, cognitive deficits, loss of balance, and memory defects?

A. <10 μg/L.
B. 10–60 μg/L.
C. 61–100 μg/L.
D. 101–200 μg/L.
E. >200 μg/L.

22.3 Common sources of lead exposure include all of the following *except*

A. Pesticides.
B. Battery production.
C. Printing.
D. Soldering.
E. Welding.

22.4 In a study conducted by Min (1986), which of the following psychiatric symptoms was found in the majority of patients who exhibited the delayed syndrome associated with carbon monoxide intoxication?

A. Depressed mood.
B. Delusions.
C. Echolalia.
D. Apathy.
E. Elated mood.

22.5 Which of the following herbal preparations is frequently used as a sedative?

A. Cola nut.
B. Kava.
C. Valerian.
D. Yohimbine.
E. Peyote.

22.6 Nerve agents are particularly potent organophosphates used for chemical warfare. What is their mechanism of action?

A. They act at the membrane level, particularly on sodium channels.
B. They inactivate the enzyme acetylcholinesterase.
C. They produce a marked loss of neurons in the hippocampus and amygdaloid nucleus.
D. They combine with hemoglobin in the blood.
E. They produce a primary axonal neuropathy.

CHAPTER 23

Neuropsychiatric Aspects of Ethanol and Other Chemical Dependencies

Select the single best response for each question.

23.1 Opiate dependence mechanisms at the level of the locus coeruleus (LC) help explain the physiological effects of these substances. Which of the following statements concerning the LC's role in opiate dependence/withdrawal is *false?*

A. Overactivation of the LC is necessary and sufficient to produce behavioral signs of opiate withdrawal.
B. The action of the α_1-adrenergic blocker clonidine mimics the effects of morphine on the LC.
C. Extrinsic activation of the LC involves excitatory glutamatergic input from the nucleus paragigantocellularis.
D. Intrinsic activation of the LC includes adaptations in opioid receptor–coupled signal transduction.
E. The LC contains the major noradrenergic nucleus in the brain.

23.2 Which of the following statements regarding the intrinsic locus coeruleus (LC) mechanism of opiate dependence is *true?*

A. Acute opiate inhibition of the LC neurons involves inhibition of the G protein–activated inward-rectifying K^+ (GIRK) channel.
B. Acute opiate inhibition of the LC neurons involves activation of inward Na^+ current.
C. Only GIRK channel effects are mediated by pertussis toxin–sensitive G proteins.
D. G proteins inhibit the GIRK channel via an indirect mechanism.
E. G protein–mediated inhibition of cyclic adenosine monophosphate (cAMP) formation influences the Na^+ current.

23.3 The mesolimbic dopamine system is involved in the reinforcing properties of several substances of abuse. However, one group of abused substances produces behavioral reinforcement independently of the dopamine system, by acting on receptors in the nucleus accumbens and other regions. Which of the following substances produces reinforcement independent of the dopamine system?

A. Opiates.
B. Psychostimulants.
C. Cannabinoids.
D. Ethanol.
E. Nicotine.

23.4 "Cross-priming," wherein dosing of one group of substances leads to increased use of another class of abusable drugs, is thought to be mediated by the mesolimbic dopamine system. Cross-priming has been clearly demonstrated for which two groups of drugs?

A. Cannabinoids and psychostimulants.
B. Cannabinoids and alcohol.
C. Nicotine and hallucinogens.
D. Opiates and alcohol.
E. Opiates and psychostimulants.

23.5 "Stress-induced" relapse into drug-seeking behavior has been studied in both animals and human subjects. Which of the following statements is *true*?

A. In animals, stress-related heroin relapse requires physiological dependence.
B. Stress-induced dopamine release in the nucleus accumbens correlates with relapse into heroin-seeking behavior.
C. Stress-induced relapse into drug use is completely attenuated with dopamine antagonists.
D. Stress attenuates release of corticotropin-releasing factor (CRF), which correlates with opiate relapse.
E. Corticosterone infusion blocks drug-seeking relapse.

23.6 What is the presumed neurochemical action of hallucinogens?

A. Stimulation of monoamine release.
B. Antagonist at *N*-methyl-D-aspartate (NMDA) glutamate receptors.
C. Antagonism of 5-hydroxytryptamine 2A (5-HT_{2A}) serotonin receptors.
D. Partial agonism at 5-hydroxytryptamine 1A (5-HT_{1A}) serotonin receptors.
E. Partial agonism at 5-HT_{2A} serotonin receptors.

23.7 "Altered physiological state that causes a withdrawal syndrome when drug taking ceases" is the definition of which of the following?

A. Tolerance.
B. Sensitization.
C. Dependence.
D. Reinforcement.
E. Addiction.

23.8 Mechanisms of dopamine-induced relapse depend on an understanding of different dopamine receptor subtypes and their effects. Which of the following statements is *true*?

A. Dopamine_1 (D_1)–like (D_1 and D_5) receptors are negatively coupled to adenylyl cyclase.
B. Dopamine_2 (D_2)–like (D_2, D_3, and D_4) receptors are positively coupled to adenylyl cyclase.
C. In the nucleus accumbens (NAc), activation of D_1-like receptors produces relapse to cocaine use in rats.
D. D_1-like receptors are responsible for priming effects in the NAc.
E. D_1-like receptor activation abolishes the ability of cocaine to induce relapse.

23.9 Which of the following substances causes decreased dendritic arborizations and decreased terminal dendritic spine density in the nucleus accumbens (NAc)?

A. Cocaine.
B. Amphetamine.
C. Nicotine.
D. Morphine.
E. None of the above.

CHAPTER 24

Neuropsychiatric Aspects of Dementias Associated With Motor Dysfunction

Select the single best response for each question.

24.1 Which of the following degenerative dementias with motor involvement is autosomal recessively inherited?

A. Huntington's disease.
B. Parkinson's disease.
C. Friedreich's ataxia.
D. Frontotemporal dementia.
E. Wilson's disease.

24.2 All of the following psychiatric disorders have been described in the literature as common comorbid conditions in Huntington's disease *except*

A. Schizophreniform disorder.
B. Intermittent explosive disorder.
C. Major depression.
D. Obsessive-compulsive disorder.
E. Bipolar disorder.

24.3 The psychiatric disorder most commonly found in patients with Parkinson's disease is

A. Psychosis.
B. Affective disorder.
C. Obsessive-compulsive disorder.
D. Generalized anxiety disorder.
E. Intermittent explosive disorder.

24.4 All of the following are clinical characteristics of diffuse Lewy body disease *except*

A. Dementia.
B. Attentional impairment.
C. Apathy.
D. Parkinsonism.
E. Fluctuations in cognitive functioning.

24.5 Which of the following clinical findings is helpful in distinguishing progressive supranuclear palsy (PSP) from Parkinson's disease?

A. Vertical eye movement abnormalities.
B. Dementia.
C. Stable gait.
D. Postural stability.
E. Axial parkinsonism with tremor.

24.6 In Wilson's disease, which brain structure degenerates in association with abnormalities in liver function?

A. Thalamus.
B. Hippocampus.
C. Amygdala.
D. Basal ganglia.
E. Corpus callosum.

CHAPTER 25

Neuropsychiatric Aspects of Alzheimer's Disease and Other Dementing Illnesses

Select the single best response for each question.

25.1 The Neuropsychiatric Inventory (NPI) completed by the caregivers of patients with mild cognitive impairment (MCI) can quantify the psychiatric comorbidity of this particular cognitive disorder. All of the following symptoms are common in MCI *except*

A. Euphoria.
B. Dysphoria.
C. Apathy.
D. Irritability.
E. Anxiety.

25.2 Alzheimer's disease is the most common dementia in the United States. As this disease progresses, a series of neurobehavioral symptoms are encountered. Which of the following symptoms develop after significant disease progression, rather than early in the course of the disease?

A. Deficient verbal and visual encoding.
B. Impaired delayed recall.
C. Concrete thinking.
D. Mild anomia.
E. Transcortical sensory aphasia.

25.3 Alzheimer's disease is associated with many behavioral symptoms, all of which can contribute significantly to functional impairment. Which of the following is the most common neuropsychiatric symptom in Alzheimer's disease?

A. Depressed mood.
B. Anxiety.
C. Apathy.
D. Irritability.
E. Psychosis.

25.4 The neuropathology of Alzheimer's disease features neuritic plaques. These plaques are deposited in different areas of cortical tissue in a progressive way. What is the site of the first deposition of plaques?

A. Frontal association cortex.
B. Parietal cortex.
C. Perirhinal cortex.
D. Temporo-occipital association cortex.
E. Entorhinal cortex.

25.5 Which medication for Alzheimer's disease blocks butyrylcholinesterase as well as acetylcholinesterase?

A. Memantine.
B. Rivastigmine.
C. Galantamine.
D. Tacrine.
E. Donepezil.

25.6 In 2005, the Expert Consensus Panel for Dementia published guidelines for treatment of psychiatric comorbidity in dementia. Which of the following was recommended as a first-line treatment for insomnia in dementia?

A. Risperidone.
B. Quetiapine.
C. Olanzapine.
D. Clonazepam.
E. Mirtazapine.

25.7 Dementia with Lewy bodies (DLB) can be distinguished from Alzheimer's disease (AD) on clinical grounds. Cognitive symptoms that are more common and severe in DLB than AD include all of the following *except*

A. Attentional deficits.
B. Visual hallucinations.
C. Cognitive fluctuations.
D. Fluctuating alertness with episodes of delirium.
E. Memory impairment.

25.8 Which of the following atypical antipsychotics is the preferred agent for treatment of hallucinations in dementia with Lewy bodies (DLB)?

A. Clozapine.
B. Olanzapine.
C. Quetiapine.
D. Risperidone.
E. None of the above.

25.9 Which of the following is *not* a feature of primary progressive aphasia?

A. Early prominent language impairment.
B. Dysfluent and agrammatic speech.
C. Early loss of language comprehension.
D. Anomia.
E. Phonemic paraphasic errors.

25.10 Vascular dementia (VaD) of the multi-infarct type is another common dementia. The constellation of cognitive symptoms in VaD suggests a subcortical pattern of deficits. All of the following deficits are typical of VaD *except*

A. Psychomotor slowing.
B. Dysexecutive symptoms.
C. Poor encoding of memory with adequate retrieval.
D. Impaired attention.
E. Poor set shifting.

25.11 Delusional misidentification syndromes occur mostly later in the disease course of dementia. Which of the following syndromes involves a conviction that a physical location has been duplicated?

A. Capgras' syndrome.
B. Fregoli's syndrome.
C. Foley's syndrome.
D. Doppelganger.
E. Reduplicative paramnesia.

C H A P T E R 2 6

Neuropsychiatric Aspects of Schizophrenia

Select the single best response for each question.

26.1 In a long-term follow-up study of patients with schizophrenia (the Vermont study), many of these patients, after 10 years of follow-up and approximately 15–20 years of illness, showed

A. A marked deterioration in mental functioning.
B. No psychotic symptoms.
C. A poor level of overall functioning, especially those over 50 years of age.
D. A deteriorating long-term course.
E. Little heterogeneity in outcome.

26.2 Which of the following candidate genes implicated in schizophrenia has also been associated with velocardiofacial syndrome?

A. Dystrobrevin binding protein-1 (*DTNBP1*).
B. Neuregulin-1 (*NRG1*).
C. Catechol-O-methyltransferase (COMT).
D. Disrupted-in-schizophrenia-1 and -2 (*DISC1* and *DISC2*).
E. Metabotropic glutamate receptor-3 (*GRM3*).

26.3 Magnetic resonance imaging (MRI) studies of the brains of patients with schizophrenia have revealed a volume decrease in all of the following brain structures *except*

A. Hippocampus.
B. Amygdala.
C. Parahippocampal gyrus.
D. Superior temporal gyrus.
E. Caudate nucleus.

26.4 A number of neurotransmitters have been implicated in schizophrenia. Phencyclidine (PCP) and ketamine cause a schizophrenic-like reaction in humans and affect which of the following neurotransmitters?

A. Dopamine.
B. Serotonin.
C. Nicotine.
D. Glutamine.
E. Acetylcholine.

26.5 The MATRICS (measurement and treatment research to improve cognition in schizophrenia) program was developed to identify potential molecular targets to treat cognitive deficits in schizophrenia (Geyer and Tamminga 2004). The molecular targets identified as having the greatest promise to improve cognition include all of the following *except*

A. Dopamine$_1$ (D_1) receptor.
B. Dopamine$_2$ (D_2) receptor.
C. α_7 Nicotinic receptor.
D. Muscarinic receptor.
E. *N*-methyl-D-aspartate (NMDA) receptor.

26.6 Positron emission tomography (PET) scanning in hallucinating persons with schizophrenia has provided clues to the anatomic structures that may be involved in a "psychosis neural circuit." The proposed psychosis circuit consists of all of the following structures *except*

A. Amygdala.
B. Medial prefrontal cortex.
C. Thalamus.
D. Anterior hippocampus.
E. Anterior cingulate.

CHAPTER 27

Neuropsychiatric Aspects of Mood Disorders

Select the single best response for each question.

27.1 Specific types of cognitive deficits are seen in mood disorders. All of the following cognitive impairments are common in depressed patients *except*

A. Slowed thought process.
B. Impaired attention.
C. Impaired concentration.
D. Language impairment.
E. Executive function impairment.

27.2 The neurochemical changes that occur in depression can affect several neurotransmitter systems. Depression is associated with all of the following neurochemical alterations *except*

A. Lower levels of cerebrospinal fluid (CSF) serotonin metabolites.
B. Decreased serotonin transporter binding.
C. Serotonin receptor abnormalities.
D. Decreased CSF homovanillic acid.
E. Increased dopamine transporter activity.

27.3 The neurobiology of depression as currently modeled involves several cortical and subcortical structures. All of the following cortical structures are thought to have a major role in depression *except*

A. Prefrontal cortex.
B. Anterior cingulate cortex.
C. Subgenual cingulate cortex.
D. Medial temporal cortex.
E. Occipital cortex.

27.4 The effect of depression on sleep patterns offers clues to understanding the neurobiology of depression. Which is the best-studied and most reproducible sleep electroencephalography (EEG) finding in depressed patients?

A. Reduced rapid eye movement (REM) latency.
B. Prolonged sleep latency.
C. Decreased slow-wave sleep.
D. Increased time in REM sleep.
E. Decreased time in non-REM sleep.

27.5 In the neural network model of depression presented in the chapter, distinct neural systems are associated with specific functions (and therefore associated with underlying symptom clusters). Cognitive, psychomotor, and sensory processing are associated with all of the following structures *except*

A. Amygdala.
B. Dorsal prefrontal cortex.
C. Dorsal anterior cingulate cortex.
D. Parietal cortex.
E. Hippocampus.

27.6 Correctly diagnosing a mood disorder in neuropsychiatric patients can be difficult, because symptoms of the neurological illness may mimic or mask the symptoms of mood disturbance. Mood symptoms less likely to be independently associated with the underlying neurological illness than with a primary mood disorder include all of the following *except*

A. Apathy.
B. Mood disturbance with consonant affect.
C. Anhedonia.
D. Excessive guilt.
E. Suicidality.

CHAPTER 28

Neuropsychiatric Aspects of Anxiety Disorders

Select the single best response for each question.

28.1 Various neuroanatomical models have been proposed for selected anxiety disorders. Which anxiety disorder is believed to be associated with increased activity in the ventromedial cortico-striatal-thalamic-cortical (CSTC) circuit?

A. Generalized anxiety disorder.
B. Obsessive-compulsive disorder (OCD).
C. Panic disorder.
D. Posttraumatic stress disorder.
E. Social anxiety disorder.

28.2 Neuroanatomical models of panic disorder emphasize the involvement of a number of brain structures and pathways. Which brain structure is believed to play a central role in conditioned fear and anxiety?

A. Thalamus.
B. Caudate.
C. Locus coeruleus.
D. Amygdala.
E. Periaqueductal gray.

28.3 Many brain structures are involved in fear and anxiety. Which of the following structures has the highest concentration of noradrenergic-producing neurons in the brain?

A. Thalamus.
B. Hypothalamus.
C. Locus coeruleus.
D. Amygdala.
E. Periaqueductal gray.

28.4 Features of current neuroanatomical models of posttraumatic stress disorder (PTSD) include all of the following *except*

A. The amygdalothalamic pathways are involved in the rapid, automatic processing of incoming information.
B. There is hyperactivation of the amygdala.
C. The hippocampus is involved in remembering the context of traumatic memories
D. The amygdala sends afferents to the hypothalamus and brain stem nuclei.
E. There is increased activity in certain frontal cortical areas such as Broca's area.

28.5 In a study examining the role of various neurochemical circuits in social anxiety disorder, investigators concluded that patients with social anxiety disorder may exhibit selective supersensitivity of which of the following circuits?

A. Serotonergic.
B. Dopaminergic.
C. Nicotinic.
D. Noradrenergic.
E. Cholinergic.

CHAPTER 29

Neuropsychiatric Disorders of Childhood and Adolescence

Select the single best response for each question.

29.1 The emergence of lateralization and hemispheric asymmetry are important to neurobehavioral development. All of the following statements are true *except*

A. Lateralization is largely established by age 5 years.
B. Differential development of the two hemispheres in early growth is due to delayed myelination of the corpus callosum.
C. In early development, the left hemisphere develops more rapidly than the right, due to its usual dominance.
D. The right hemisphere accelerates its development between the ages of 3 and 6 years.
E. Gray matter density tends to be greater in the right posterior temporal regions than the left.

29.2 Psychiatric comorbidity in attention-deficit/hyperactivity disorder (ADHD) often complicates this already difficult-to-manage disorder. Which of the following statements is *true?*

A. Conduct disorder occurs in 20%–40% of ADHD cases.
B. Abused children with both posttraumatic stress disorder (PTSD) and ADHD have the same degree of motor hyperactivity as do children with classic ADHD alone.
C. Thyroid hormone resistance is a common cause of ADHD.
D. A high incidence of ADHD is found with girls, but not boys, with Tourette's syndrome.
E. ADHD-type symptoms may indicate genetic risk in schizophrenia pedigrees.

29.3 Imaging studies have helped to delineate a constellation of brain regions involved in attention-deficit/hyperactivity disorder (ADHD). Which of the following is the most consistent neuroanatomical finding in ADHD subjects relative to non-ADHD controls?

A. Decreased size of the caudate.
B. Increased size of the frontal cortex.
C. Increased size of the posterior portion of the corpus callosum.
D. Decreased size of the cerebellar vermis.
E. Increased size of the anterior portion of the corpus callosum.

29.4 Psychostimulant medications remain the cornerstone of attention-deficit/hyperactivity disorder (ADHD) treatment. Common side effects of psychostimulants include all of the following *except*

A. Anorexia.
B. Irritability.
C. Dysphoria.
D. Tics and other stereotypic movements.
E. Insomnia.

29.5 Tic disorders are often comorbid with obsessive-compulsive disorder (OCD). However, the OCD symptoms in tic disorder patients often differ from the symptoms in patients with classic OCD. All of the following statements are true *except*

A. OCD is seen in approximately 10% of Tourette's syndrome patients.
B. OCD symptoms usually appear 1–2 years before simple tics in these patients.
C. Tic-related OCD has an earlier onset than does classic OCD.
D. Tic-related OCD features more ritualized touching and tapping than does classic OCD.
E. Tic-related OCD has a less favorable response to selective serotonin reuptake inhibitors (SSRIs) and a more favorable response to antipsychotic augmentation compared with classic OCD.

29.6 Fragile X syndrome, the most common known inherited cause of mental retardation, is often associated with autism-spectrum behaviors. Which of the following symptoms is *not* characteristic of fragile X syndrome?

A. Social withdrawal and reduced caregiver attachment.
B. Gaze avoidance.
C. Hand flapping.
D. Tactile defensiveness.
E. Perseveration.

29.7 Prader-Willi syndrome is a genetic form of mental retardation characterized by specific morphological and behavioral abnormalities. Which of the following features is *not* characteristic of this illness?

A. Growth retardation.
B. Precocious sexual development.
C. Obesity.
D. Hyperphagia.
E. Short stature.

29.8 Seizure disorders in children are a vexing source of neurological and psychiatric symptoms. A childhood seizure that features alterations in consciousness; auras of unpleasant odors, tastes, and sensations; and simple, repetitive, and purposeless automatisms is classified as what type of seizure?

A. Simple partial seizure.
B. Partial sensory seizure.
C. Rolandic epilepsy.
D. Complex partial seizure.
E. Frontal lobe epilepsy.

29.9 Pediatric autoimmune neuropsychiatric disorders associated with streptococcal infection (PANDAS) presents a fascinating model of infectious disease–associated neuropsychiatric illness. The Swedo criteria for PANDAS include all of the following *except*

A. Presence of obsessive-compulsive disorder (OCD) and/or tic disorder.
B. Onset before age 7 years.
C. Episodic course of symptom severity.
D. Association with group A β-hemolytic streptococcal (GABHS) infection.
E. Association with neurological abnormalities.

CHAPTER 30

Intracellular and Intercellular Principles of Pharmacotherapy for Neuropsychiatric Disorders

Select the single best response for each question.

30.1 Which of the following statements concerning glia (astrocytes) is *false*?

A. Glia protect neurons by limiting synaptic levels of glutamate.
B. Glia play a prominent role in recycling and conserving glutamate.
C. Glia possess membrane transporters for glutamate.
D. Glutamate is metabolized to γ-aminobutyric acid (GABA) in the glial cell.
E. Glutamate is involved in opening of specific calcium channels that allow influx of calcium ions into neurons.

30.2 Astroglia play a pivotal role in the regulation of brain physiology and neuronal activity via the nitric oxide (NO) pathway. Which of the following is the precursor of NO?

A. Glutamate.
B. γ-Aminobutyric acid (GABA).
C. L-Arginine.
D. Glutamine.
E. Glutamine synthetase.

30.3 Chemical transmission requires the presence of several elements to operate effectively. These elements may focus on the presynaptic, synaptic, or postsynaptic portion of the neuron. Which of the following elements is required for chemical transmission at the synaptic level?

A. Enzymes for neurotransmitter synthesis.
B. Coupler proteins.
C. Mechanism for neurotransmitter storage.
D. Neurotransmitter receptors to initiate response.
E. Mechanism for terminating neurotransmitter action.

30.4 Which of the following receptor types has seven transmembrane sections of the protein with extracellular and intracellular loops that serve as neurotransmitter binding sites?

A. Receptors that form ion channels.
B. G protein–coupled receptors.
C. Receptors that act on allosteric sites.
D. Steroid transcription factor binding receptors.
E. Receptors that synthesize components of synaptic transmission.

30.5 At this time, only one known psychotherapeutic agent likely has its mechanism of action in a second-messenger system. This agent is…

A. Lithium.
B. Haloperidol.
C. Chlorpromazine.
D. Carbamazepine.
E. Clozapine.

30.6 Which of the following statements concerning nitric oxide (NO) is *true*?

A. NO is stored in presynaptic nerve endings.
B. NO interacts with specific receptors.
C. NO's influence is synaptic in nature.
D. NO is not a gas in the central nervous system.
E. NO is synthesized on demand.

30.7 Which of the following neurotransmitter types uses only cyclic adenosine monophosphate (cAMP) as its messenger system?

A. Glycine.
B. Angiotensin.
C. Dopamine.
D. Cortisol.
E. Glutamate.

CHAPTER 31

Psychopharmacological Treatments for Patients With Neuropsychiatric Disorders

Select the single best response for each question.

31.1 Depression and apathy are common complications of neuropsychiatric illness and require clinical subtlety in their management. Among the following antidepressant agents, which is most likely to be useful for apathy with depressed mood?

A. Amitriptyline.
B. Selective serotonergic and noradrenergic reuptake inhibitors (SNRIs).
C. Doxepin.
D. Nonselective monoamine oxidase inhibitors (MAOIs).
E. Bupropion.

31.2 Psychosis complicating neuropsychiatric illness can be seen in a number of syndromes but is generally less common than mood disorders. Which of the following is *least* likely to be associated with psychosis?

A. Stroke.
B. Complex partial seizures.
C. Huntington's disease.
D. Human immunodeficiency virus (HIV) disease.
E. Late-stage Parkinson's disease.

31.3 Because of the dopamine-deficient state in Parkinson's disease, management of psychosis in this condition poses a significant risk of exacerbating motor symptoms. This can be mitigated somewhat by judicious use of atypical antipsychotics. Which of the following agents in this class is the most efficacious for psychosis in Parkinson's disease?

A. Risperidone.
B. Olanzapine.
C. Aripiprazole.
D. Ziprasidone.
E. Clozapine.

31.4 Mania, depression, and anxiety may be associated with a range of neuropsychiatric illnesses. All of the following statements are true *except*

A. Stroke is rarely associated with mania.
B. Mania is far less common in patients with traumatic brain injury (TBI) than in the general population.
C. Multiple sclerosis patients have a higher risk of mania than the general population.
D. Stroke patients with cortical lesions are more likely to have anxiety and depression than are those with subcortical lesions.
E. HIV patients have a higher risk of mania than the general population.

31.5 Lithium has been reported to have a robust effect on which particular type of mania?

A. Mania associated with human immunodeficiency virus (HIV).
B. Mania associated with traumatic brain injury (TBI).
C. Mania associated with steroid use.
D. Mania associated with Parkinson's disease.
E. Mania associated with multiple sclerosis.

31.6 β-Adrenergic blockers may be a therapeutic option in agitated states. All of the following statements are true *except*

A. Response may take up to 8 weeks.
B. Both central and peripheral β blockade may contribute to these agents' therapeutic action.
C. Secondary depression is common and often limits the use of β-blockers.
D. β-Blockers are contraindicated in chronic obstructive pulmonary disease (COPD).
E. Dosages of up to 12 mg/kg/day are recommended for propranolol.

31.7 Concerning the use of psychostimulants to treat cognitive impairment, which of the following statements is *false*?

A. Stimulants have been shown to improve neuropsychological testing performance in HIV disease.
B. Stimulants are generally well tolerated in neurological patients.
C. Stimulants may enhance cortical recovery.
D. Stimulants lower the seizure threshold, a major limitation in their utility.
E. Stimulants may increase delusional thought content.

CHAPTER 32

Psychotherapy for Patients With Neuropsychiatric Disorders

Select the single best response for each question.

32.1 Because patients with neuropsychiatric disorders may exhibit impairments in selected hierarchical capacities, psychiatrists will need to adapt their psychotherapeutic techniques to assist the patient in managing these impairments. By adopting a reassuring manner, avoiding overstimulation, and limiting the time of visit, the psychiatrist will address which capacity that may be impaired?

A. Consciousness.
B. Attention.
C. Retention.
D. Orientation.
E. Recognition.

32.2 Patients with neuropsychiatric disorders may misidentify others. Eight variant forms of misidentification have been described. What is the appropriate term to describe the form of misidentification in which a patient believes that a familiar person has assumed another bodily form?

A. Capgras' delusions, "Body Snatchers" type.
B. Intermetamorphosis.
C. Fregoli type.
D. Subjective doubles, Capgras type.
E. Reverse subjective doubles, autoscopic type.

32.3 Traumatic brain injury results principally from vehicular accidents, falls, acts of violence, and sports injuries. Which population age group is at highest risk of such injury?

A. 0–5 years.
B. 6–14 years.
C. 15–24 years.
D. 25–60 years.
E. 61–74 years.

32.4 Traumatic brain injury (TBI) will have a profound effect upon families. Which of the following statements concerning the impact of TBI on families is *true?*

A. Wives and mothers of TBI patients may experience increases in anxiety and social dysfunction, but the symptoms are brief, usually lasting less than 6 months.
B. The physical deficits from TBI are more troubling than the cognitive and affective changes.
C. The father of a TBI patient is the parent most likely to be able to handle stress.
D. Mothers of TBI patients usually assume the role of case managers.
E. When TBI patients are hospitalized, the hospital staff is often a source of support to the family, especially when conflicts arise.

32.5 Which of the following statements concerning treatment considerations in early Parkinson's disease is *true?*

A. During the early phases of the illness, patients should be exposed to patients with advanced stages of the illness so they will know what to expect.
B. The patient's significant other should be referred to as the caregiver.
C. Demands from the patient for secrecy of the diagnosis are often indicative of paranoid ideation.
D. Psychotherapy is of little value in managing tremor and bradykinesia.
E. During the early stages, patients should practice being more facially demonstrative.

32.6 In managing patients with Huntington's disease, psychiatrists should

A. Participate in denial of transmissibility.
B. Discuss fantasies that the disease is a punishment.
C. Avoid addressing family ambivalence about preserving life in a downhill course.
D. Refrain from pointing out that preservation of recognition may lead to depression.
E. Resist the temptation to interpret blame of the gene-donating parent.

CHAPTER 33

Cognitive Rehabilitation and Behavior Therapy for Patients With Neuropsychiatric Disorders

Select the single best response for each question.

33.1 Cognitive rehabilitation requires tailoring the therapy to the patient's specific deficits. In the Orientation Remedial Program, all of the following task areas are included *except*

A. Attending and reacting to environmental signals.
B. Timing responses in relation to environmental signals.
C. Being actively vigilant.
D. Estimating time.
E. Responding on the basis of simple rhythms.

33.2 Steps in the "PQRST" method for remembering written information include all of the following *except*

A. **P**review of the information.
B. Form **Q**uestions about the information.
C. **R**ehearse responses.
D. **S**tate questions.
E. **T**est for retention.

33.3 Patients with frontal lobe impairments often have different rehabilitative needs than those with temporal lobe deficits. Which of the following symptoms is characteristic of temporal, rather than frontal, lobe symptoms?

A. Heightened interpersonal sensitivity and paranoid ideation.
B. Social disinhibition.
C. Reduced attention.
D. Distractibility.
E. Impaired judgment.

33.4 Various interventions are used to address dysfunctional behaviors observed in individuals with neurological impairment. A behavioral approach wherein there is reinforcement of a behavior inconsistent with the target problem behavior is called

A. Extinction.
B. Positive reinforcement.
C. Negative reinforcement.
D. Differential reinforcement of other behavior.
E. Antecedent management.

CHAPTER 1

Cellular and Molecular Biology of the Neuron

Select the single best response for each question.

1.1 Glial cells are divided into three classes (astrocytes, oligodendrocytes, and microglia) with various different neurophysiological functions. All of the following are functions of astrocytes *except*

A. Structural "scaffolding" of the brain.
B. Formation of the blood-brain barrier.
C. Guidance of neuronal migration during brain development.
D. Cell-cell signaling, often over long distances.
E. Production of the myelin sheath.

The correct response is option E.

The myelin sheath, which speeds conduction of the action potential along axons, is produced by oligodendrocytes.

Astrocytes have three traditional functions: they provide the scaffolding of the brain, form the blood-brain barrier, and guide neuronal migration during development. Evidence is also accumulating that astroglial cells are more dynamic than previously suspected and are capable of cell-cell signaling over long distances. **(p. 4)**

1.2 Which of the following statements regarding the electrochemical events involved in the generation of action potentials is *false*?

A. Na^+ and Cl^- are strongly concentrated outside the neuronal cell membrane.
B. K^+ is strongly concentrated within the neuronal cell membrane.
C. At rest, voltage-gated K^+ and Cl^- channels remain closed to preserve equilibrium.
D. The baseline membrane potential is between –50 and –75 mV.
E. Depolarization is only approximately a millisecond because of time-dependent inactivation of Na^+ channels.

The correct response is option C.

At rest, K^+ and Cl^- channels are open so that K^+ and Cl^- gradients determine the membrane potential, causing the cell to be negative inside by about –50 to –75 mV.

The ability of neurons to generate an action potential derives from the presence of strong ionic gradients across the membrane: Na^+ and Cl^- are highly concentrated outside the membrane, while K^+ is highly concentrated inside. The membrane potential stays depolarized for only about a millisecond, because Na^+ channels then show a time-dependent inactivation. **(pp. 6–7; Figure 1–2)**

1.3 Which of the following statements regarding the neurophysiology of signaling between neurons is *true*?

A. Chemical synapses are formed by gap junctions.
B. Most central nervous system (CNS) synaptic connections are mediated by electrical synapses.
C. Glial cells are connected by gap junctions.
D. Chemical synapses are limited in that they do not allow for signal modulation.
E. Chemical synapses are solely excitatory.

The correct response is option C.

Glial cells are connected by gap junctions, which link these cells into large syncytia, providing avenues for intercellular propagation of chemical signals mediated by small molecules and ions, such as Ca^{2+}.

Electrical synapses are formed by gap junctions. Most CNS synaptic connections are mediated by chemical neurotransmitters. Although chemical synapses are slower than electrical ones, they allow for signal amplification, may be inhibitory as well as excitatory, are susceptible to a wide range of modulation, and can modulate the activities of other cells through the release of transmitters activating second-messenger cascades. **(p. 10)**

1.4 The two major classes of neurotransmitters are small-molecule transmitters (which mediate fast synaptic transmission and are stored in small, clear vesicles) and neuropeptides (which modulate synaptic transmission and are stored in large, dense-core vesicles). All of the following are classified as small-molecule transmitters *except*

A. Opioids.
B. γ-Aminobutyric acid (GABA).
C. Acetylcholine.
D. Serotonin.
E. Dopamine.

The correct response is option A.

Opioids are classified as neuropeptides, as are somatostatin, the hypothalamic-releasing hormones, endorphins, and enkephalins.

GABA, glycine, acetylcholine, serotonin, dopamine, norepinephrine, epinephrine, and histamine are classified as small-molecule transmitters. **(p. 10)**

1.5 The process of neurotransmitter release involves several sequential steps. Potent neurotoxins, such as botulinum and tetanus toxin, exert their effects by blocking which step in this cascade of events?

A. Vesicle docking in active zones.
B. Priming.
C. Fusion/exocytosis.
D. Endocytosis.
E. Synaptic vesicle refilling.

The correct response is option B.

Botulinum and tetanus toxin block synaptic transmission by proteolysis of key molecules involved in priming.

Neurotransmitter release involves a six-step cycle: 1) vesicles dock at active zones before exocytotic release. 2) Priming occurs, whereby vesicles become ready to respond to increases in intracellular Ca^{2+}. 3) Triggered by an influx in Ca^{2+}, fusion/exocytosis then occurs in less than a millisecond, releasing the neurotransmitter into the synaptic cleft. 4) Endocytosis recovers the synaptic vesicle membrane. 5) Synaptic vesicles are refilled with neurotransmitter, driven by an acidic intravesicular gradient. 6) The filled synaptic vesicles are transported back to the active zone to complete the cycle. **(p. 11)**

1.6 The process of neural development begins with proliferative zones, which line the lumen of the developing ventricular system. All of the following statements regarding neuronal development and migration are true *except*

A. The ventricular zone (VZ), adjacent to the ventricular lumen, contains pseudostratified columnar epithelial cells, now called radial glial cells.
B. A second proliferative zone, the subventricular zone (SVZ), appears just above the VZ.
C. VZ precursor cells are the source of SVZ progenitor cells.
D. SVZ cells are bipolar and maintain physical contact with the pial and ventricular surfaces.
E. Radial glial cells can generate neurons before transforming into astrocytes.

The correct response is option D.

SVZ cells are multipolar, they do not maintain contact with the pial and ventricular surfaces as do radial glial cells, they do not undergo interkinetic nuclear migration as they proceed through the cell cycle, and they divide away from the ventricular lumen. **(pp. 23–24)**

1.7 In the development of synapses, there are three classes of signals that regulate synaptic formation: adhesion molecules, diffusible molecules, and molecules secreted from glial cells. Which of the following is considered to be one of the diffusible molecules?

A. Brain-derived neurotrophic factor (BDNF).
B. Integrins.
C. Nectins.
D. Cadherins.
E. Ephrins.

The correct response is option A.

BDNF and members of the Wnt and TGFβ families are considered diffusible molecules.

Integrins, nectins, cadherins, ephrins, neural cell adhesion molecules (NCAMs), neurexin–neuroligin, and synaptic adhesion molecules (SynCAMs) are adhesion molecules. **(pp. 28, 30)**

1.8 Apoptosis is a genetically programmed mechanism of cell death that is crucial to brain development. Which of the following is *not* a component of apoptosis?

A. Cytoplasmic shrinkage.
B. Chromatin condensation.
C. Degradation of neuronal DNA.
D. Dependence on RNA and protein synthesis.
E. An active inflammatory response.

The correct response is option E.

Apoptosis, unlike necrosis, does not stimulate an inflammatory response. Apoptosis, characterized by cytoplasmic shrinkage, chromatin condensation, and degradation of DNA into oligonucleosomal fragments, is an active process that requires RNA and protein synthesis. **(p. 30)**

1.9 Glutamate-mediated excitotoxicity is an important process affecting many neuropsychiatric illnesses. Which of the following statements regarding this important mechanism is *false?*

A. Excitotoxicity is mediated by Na^+ entry via α-amino-3-hydroxy-5-methylisoxazole-4-propionic acid (AMPA) channels.
B. Excitotoxicity is the probable mechanism in neuronal loss in stroke.
C. Neuronal depolarization evokes increases in glutamate release.
D. Sustained entry of Ca^{2+} into cells through AMPA channels results in delayed excitotoxicity.
E. Injured neurons show excess levels of intracellular Ca^{2+}.

The correct response is option D.

Sustained Ca^{2+} entry through *N*-methyl-D-aspartate (NMDA) receptor channels causes a delayed mode of excitotoxicity that kills neurons, probably by activation of intracellular proteases and/or generation of free radicals, including nitric oxide (NO).

Excitotoxicity appears to be mediated acutely by Na^+ through AMPA channels, which leads to neuronal swelling, resulting in brain edema. Excitotoxicity probably underlies neuronal loss in strokes, status epilepticus, hypoglycemia, and head trauma. These brain insults are linked in that all lead to neuronal depolarization, which results in excessive electrical activity, evoking excessive increases in glutamate release. Injured neurons show increased intracellular levels of Ca^{2+}, and excitatory amino acid antagonists, especially those blocking NMDA receptors or channels, prevent or dramatically reduce neuronal loss in these conditions. **(p. 34)**

CHAPTER 2

Functional Neuroanatomy: Neuropsychological Correlates of Cortical and Subcortical Damage

Select the single best response for each question.

2.1 The left and right hemispheres of the human brain differ in several fundamental ways. All of the following statements concerning lateral specialization are true *except*

A. In the vast majority of people, the left hemisphere is specialized for language and for processing verbally coded information.
B. The right hemisphere processes nonverbal information such as visual patterns or auditory signals.
C. The left hemisphere is specialized for the perception of our bodies in space.
D. The right hemisphere is dedicated to the mapping of feeling states.
E. The left hemisphere is involved in the processing of verbal information apprehended through either auditory or visual channels.

The correct response is option C.

The right hemisphere is specialized for the perception of our bodies in space.

In the vast majority of adults, the left side of the brain is specialized for language and for processing verbally coded information. This is true of nearly all (88%) right-handed individuals, the majority (75%) of left-handed persons, and 43% of mixed-handed persons. Thus, verbal information learned through either the auditory or visual channel is processed preferentially by the left hemisphere. The right hemisphere processes nonverbal information such as complex visual patterns or auditory signals that are not coded in verbal form, and it is also dedicated to the mapping of feeling states. **(pp. 46–47)**

2.2 There are several major subdivisions of the temporal lobe. Where is the hippocampus located?

A. Nonmesial portion of the temporal lobe.
B. The mesial temporal lobe.
C. Posterior portion of the superior temporal gyrus.
D. Temporal pole.
E. Inferotemporal region.

The correct response is option B.

The mesial temporal lobe includes the hippocampus, the amygdala, the entorhinal and perirhinal cortices, and a portion of the anterior parahippocampal gyrus.

The nonmesial portion of the temporal lobe includes the temporal pole, the inferotemporal region, and the region of transition between the posterior temporal lobe and the inferior occipital lobe. The posterior portion of the superior temporal gyrus forms the heart of what is traditionally known as Wernicke's area. **(pp. 48, 50 [Figure 2–4])**

2.3 With respect to the nature of amnesia associated with hippocampal damage, all of the following statements are true *except*

A. Neuropsychological findings have demonstrated selective impairments in relational memory.
B. The hippocampal system mediates long-term relational memory.
C. There is a consistent relationship between the side of the hippocampal lesion and the type of learning impairment.
D. The hippocampal system plays a role in the learning of perceptuomotor skills.
E. The hippocampal system is not the principal repository for old memories.

The correct response is option D.

The hippocampal system does not appear to play a role in the learning of perceptuomotor skills and other knowledge (referred to as *nondeclarative memory*).

Neuropsychological findings have demonstrated selected impairments in relational memory, and this has been supported by functional neuroimaging research as well. More recent work has suggested that the hippocampal system specifically mediates long-term relational memory. There is a consistent relationship between the side of the lesion and the type of learning impairment. Specifically, damage to the left hippocampal system produces an amnesic syndrome that affects verbal material but spares nonverbal material; conversely, damage to the right hippocampal system affects nonverbal material but spares verbal material. The hippocampal system is not the principal repository for old memories. **(pp. 51, 52)**

2.4 The amygdala plays an important role in

A. The recognition of emotion.
B. The classical conditioning of autonomic responses.
C. The processing of stimuli that communicate emotional significance in social situations.
D. The decision-making process.
E. All of the above.

The correct response is option E.

The amygdala is important for the recognition of emotion, especially fear; it is important for classical conditioning of autonomic responses; for processing stimuli that communicate emotional significance in social situations; and in decision making. **(p. 53)**

2.5 Optic ataxia...

A. Is a disturbance of visually guided reaching behavior.
B. Is a deficit of visual scanning.
C. Consists of an inability to direct the gaze voluntarily toward a stimulus located in the peripheral vision to bring it into central vision.
D. Is necessary for the development of visual disorientation.
E. Is characterized by patients having difficulty pointing to sound sources.

The correct response is option A.

Optic ataxia is a disturbance of visually guided reaching behavior.

Ocular apraxia is a deficit of visual scanning, which consists of the inability to direct the gaze voluntarily toward a stimulus located in the peripheral vision to bring it into central vision. Ocular apraxia is not necessary for the development of visual disorientation. In cases of optic ataxia, the patients have no difficulty pointing to sound sources. **(pp. 59–60)**

2.6 Which of the following statements concerning Wernicke's aphasia is *false*?

A. It is hallmarked by fluent, paraphasic speech.
B. Patients exhibit impaired repetition.
C. Patients' aural comprehension remains intact.
D. Patients produce speech without hesitation.
E. The phrase length and melodic contour of utterances are normal.

The correct response is option C.

Wernicke's aphasia is hallmarked by fluent, paraphasic speech, impaired repetition, and defective aural comprehension. Patients produce speech without hesitation, and the phrase length and melodic contour of utterances are normal; however, there are frequent errors in the choice of individual words used to express an idea. Phonemic and semantic paraphasias are common. Repetition of sentences is impaired and may be limited to single words. Repetition of digits is usually impaired as well. The comprehension defect can be quite severe and frequently involves both aural and written forms of language. **(p. 63)**

2.7 Which of the following statements concerning Broca's aphasia is *true*?

A. Patients have fluent speech.
B. The aphasia is characterized by long utterances.
C. There is a marked increase in the density of words per unit time.
D. Paraphasias are uncommon.
E. A defect in repetition is invariably present.

The correct response is option E.

A defect in repetition is invariably present in patients with Broca's aphasia. Most patients have defective naming and impaired writing, whereas their language comprehension is relatively preserved.

Patients with Broca's aphasia have nonfluent speech, characterized by short utterances, and show a marked decrease in the density of words per unit time. **(pp. 68, 70)**

2.8 The dorsolateral prefrontal cortex region of the brain…

A. Occupies Brodmann areas 11, 12, 25, and 32.
B. Is involved in working memory.
C. Mediates long-term storage of information.
D. May be assessed for deficits by asking the patient important historical dates in his or her life (e.g., date of birth, wedding anniversary, birthdates of children).
E. None of the above.

The correct response is option B.

The dorsolateral prefrontal region (Brodmann areas 8, 9, 10, and 46) has been linked to *working memory*, a relatively short (on the order of minutes) window of mental processing during which information is held "on-line," and operations are performed on it. In essence, working memory is a temporary storage and process system used for problem solving and other cognitive operations that take place over a limited time frame. Tests used to assess working memory include the Digit Span backwards test from the Wechsler Adult Intelligence Scale—III and the "serial 7s" test. Remembering important historical dates in one's life is a function of long-term memory, not of working memory. **(pp. 75, 76)**

2.9 The basal ganglia are a set of deep gray nuclear structures which include which of the following?

A. Lenticular nucleus.
B. Putamen.
C. Caudate nucleus.
D. Globus pallidus.
E. All of the above.

The correct response is option E.

The basal ganglia are a set of deep gray nuclear structures which include the caudate nucleus and the lenticular nucleus, which is divided into the putamen and the globus pallidus. **(p. 76)**

CHAPTER 3

Nervous, Endocrine, and Immune System Interactions in Psychiatry

Select the single best response for each question.

3.1 A major branch point in classification of immune system cells is the distinction between "lymphoid" and "myeloid" cell lines. Which of the following cell types is classified as lymphoid?

A. B cells.
B. Monocytes.
C. Neutrophils.
D. Basophils.
E. Eosinophils.

The correct response is option A.

The lymphoid cell line includes B cells, T cells, and natural killer (NK) cells.

The myeloid cell line includes monocytes and granulocytes such as neutrophils, basophils, and eosinophils. **(pp. 93–94)**

3.2 Cytokines are immune signaling factors which serve as important mediators in immunity and disease. Many of the cytokines have important relationships to psychiatric symptoms and illnesses. Which of the cytokines is produced by macrophages, fibroblasts, lymphoblastoid cells, and virally infected cells and includes in its activities the increased expression of histocompatibility molecules, induction of viral resistance, and stimulation of natural killer cells?

A. Interleukin 1.
B. Interleukin 2.
C. Interleukin 6.
D. Interferon α.
E. Interferon β.

The correct response is option D.

Interferon α is the cytokine described.

Interleukin 1 is produced by activated macrophages, B cells, neutrophils, astrocytes, and epithelial and endothelial cells; activates B cells, helper T cells, and endothelial cells; stimulates acute phase protein production; promotes inflammation and hematopoiesis; and centrally induces fever, somnolence, and anorexia.

Interleukin 2 is produced by antigen-activated T helper 1 (Th1) cells and promotes growth and differentiation of T and B lymphocytes and proliferation of natural killer (NK) cells.

Interleukin 6 is produced by T helper 2 (Th2) cells, macrophages, fibroblasts, epithelium, and adipocytes; promotes B cell growth and differentiation and antibody secretion; and stimulates hepatocytes to produce acute phase proteins.

Interferon β is produced by fibroblasts, endothelial cells, and virally infected cells, and it stimulates NK cell activity and induces resistance to virus. **(pp. 94, 95 [Table 3–1])**

3.3 The distinction between innate (or natural) immunity and acquired immunity is based on the necessity for prior exposure to the antigen. These two complementary systems are mediated by several soluble mediators. Which of the following soluble mediators is associated with innate immunity?

A. Interferon γ.
B. Interleukin 1 (IL-1).
C. Interleukin 2 (IL-2).
D. Interleukin 4 (IL-4).
E. Interleukin 10 (IL-10).

The correct response is option B.

IL-1 is a soluble mediator associated with innate immunity. Interferon γ, IL-2, IL-4, and IL-10 are associated with acquired immunity. **(pp. 94, 96 [Table 3–2])**

3.4 Acquired immunity is a complex process that follows exposure to an antigen, so that the antigen is "remembered" by the immune system. All of the following are phases in the mechanism of the acquired immune response *except*

A. Induction phase.
B. Activation phase.
C. Effector phase.
D. Memory phase.
E. Complement protein amplification phase.

The correct response is option E.

Complement protein amplification phase is not part of the acquired immune response.

Acquired immunity occurs in four phases: an "induction phase," in which an infectious agent or antigen is detected; an "activation phase," in which immune cells proliferate and mobilize; an "effector phase," in which the agent or antigen is neutralized and eliminated; and a "memory phase," in which immune cells capable of responding to reexposure to antigen are maintained in the circulation. **(pp. 97–98)**

3.5 The organism's immunological response to stress is conceptualized in both acute and chronic time frames, with some differences in immunological mediator function in these two responses. Although this work is based on animal models, the immunological response to stress may have important correlates in psychiatric illness. Which of the following changes is characteristic of *chronic* stress in laboratory animals?

A. Decreased antibody production.
B. Decreased phagocyte function.
C. Increased acute phase proteins.
D. Activation of nuclear factor–kappa B (NFkB).
E. Increased number of circulating natural killer (NK) cells.

The correct response is option A.

Decreased antibody production is characteristic of chronic stress in laboratory animals. All of the other changes listed—decreased phagocyte function, increased acute phase proteins, activation of NFkB, and increased number of circulating NK cells—are immune responses to *acute* stress. **(p. 102, Table 3–3)**

3.6 In human studies, the differentiation of acute vs. chronic stress response reveals some differences in immune functions but also some similarities. Which of the following is associated with chronic stress but not acute stress in human subjects?

A. Decreased natural killer (NK) cell activity.
B. Increased production of proinflammatory cytokines.
C. Increased white blood cell count.
D. Increased antibody titer to viruses.
E. Decreased antibody response to vaccine.

The correct response is option A.

Decreased NK cell activity is an immune response to chronic stress in humans. All of the other changes listed—increased production of proinflammatory cytokines, increased white blood cell count, increased antibody titer to viruses, and decreased antibody response to vaccine—are immune responses to acute stress. **(p. 103 [Table 3–4])**

3.7 Rheumatoid arthritis (RA) is a systemic illness with much psychiatric comorbidity in clinical practice. Which of the following statements regarding the immunological aspects of RA is *true*?

A. Rheumatoid factor (RF) positive patients show a strong association between stressful events and disease onset.
B. RA patients typically demonstrate profound increases in cortisol following surgery and other major interventions.
C. Treatment of depression in RA is associated with improved mood but no improvement in pain or physical disability.
D. In RA, both joint swelling and depression are associated with increased levels of the soluble interleukin-2 receptor (sIL-2R).
E. RA is associated with an excess of T helper 1 (Th1) cell activation.

The correct response is option E.

Rheumatoid arthritis is accompanied by an excess of Th1 cell activation.

RF-negative patients, not RF-positive ones, show higher scores on scales reporting negative life events before the onset of the disease. Patients with osteomyelitis exhibit increases in cortisol and IL-1β and IL-6 after surgery. Treatment of depression in RA, when treated with antidepressants, leads to improvements in RA-associated pain and disability. Although joint swelling has been found to correspond to increased sIL-2R levels, disturbed mood is surprisingly associated with decreased sIL-2R levels. **(pp. 107–108)**

3.8 A reported syndrome of "sickness behavior" or "neurovegetative syndrome" may be seen with the therapeutic use of cytokines that overlaps with major depression phenomenologically. There is also a "mood/cognitive" syndrome seen in these patients. This may lead to clinical ambiguity in the management of complex clinical conditions; e.g., the treatment of depression in a patient with hepatitis C who is also receiving the cytokine interferon-α. Which of the following statements regarding behavioral symptoms in interferon therapy is *true*?

A. The "mood/cognitive" syndrome occurs early in interferon-α therapy and is nonresponsive to antidepressants.
B. The "neurovegetative syndrome" usually occurs early in interferon treatment and is responsive to antidepressants.
C. The "mood/cognitive" syndrome is associated with suppression of corticotropin-releasing hormone (CRH) pathways.
D. The "mood/cognitive" syndrome is associated with normal serotonin metabolism and altered dopamine metabolism.
E. The "mood/cognitive" syndrome appears late in interferon treatment and is responsive to antidepressants.

The correct response is option E.

The "mood/cognitive" syndrome appears late during interferon-α therapy and is responsive to antidepressants. In addition, it is associated with activation of CRH pathways and altered serotonin metabolism.

The "neurovegetative syndrome" appears early during interferon treatment, is nonresponsive to antidepressants, and may be mediated by alterations in basal ganglia dopamine metabolism. **(pp. 121, 122)**

CHAPTER 4

Bedside Neuropsychiatry: Eliciting the Clinical Phenomena of Neuropsychiatric Illness

Select the single best response for each question.

4.1 Some physical anomalies are stable through childhood and give clues to abnormal neurodevelopment in adulthood. A scale that is in common use to note these anomalies is called the Waldrop scale. Which of the following minor physical anomalies is *not* included in this scale?

A. Small nails.
B. Wide-spaced eyes.
C. Adherent ear lobes.
D. Furrowed tongue.
E. Abnormal palm crease.

The correct response is option A.

Small nails is not included in the Waldrop scale.

Minor physical anomalies included in the Waldrop scale are head circumference; two or more hair whorls; fine, "electric" hair that will not comb down; wide-spaced eyes; epicanthus; adherent ear lobes; malformation or asymmetry of ears; low-seated or soft and pliable ears; high arch of palate; furrowed tongue; geographic tongue; clinodactyly; abnormal palm crease; third toe longer than second toe; partial syndactyly; and a gap between first and second toes. **(pp. 141, 142 [Table 4–1])**

4.2 Palilalia is defined as

A. The patient's repetition of speech of another person.
B. The patient's automatic repetition of his or her own word or phrase.
C. The patient's speech marked by impulsive utterances of stereotyped or simple responses with no aphasic or echolalic features.
D. Loss of the production or recognition of affective elements of speech.
E. A disorder of fluency in which discourse, rather than purely articulation, is disturbed by a range of deficits in speech pragmatics, motor control, and attention.

The correct response is option B.

Palilalia is the automatic repetition of the patient's own words or phrases.

Echolalia is the patient's automatic repetition of the speech of another person without communicative intent or effect. Blurting is speech marked by impulsive utterances of stereotyped responses with no aphasic or echolalic features. Aprosodia is the loss of the production or recognition of affective elements of speech. And finally, cluttering is a disorder of fluency in which discourse, rather than purely articulation, is disturbed by a range of deficits in speech pragmatics, motor control, and attention. **(pp. 145–146)**

4.3 Tremors are rhythmic, regular, oscillating movements. In rest tremor, the movement is present distally when the limb is supported and relaxed; action reduces the intensity of the tremor. The most common disorder associated with this tremor is

A. Hereditary, essential tremor.
B. Anxiety.
C. Metabolic encephalopathy.
D. Medication induced (caffeine, lithium).
E. Parkinson's disease.

The correct response is option E.

Three major forms of tremor are distinguished. Parkinson's disease is the most common disorder associated with *rest tremor.* In *postural tremor,* the outstretched limb oscillates. At times, this can be better visualized by placing a piece of paper over the outstretched hand. Postural tremor is produced by anxiety, by certain drugs (e.g., caffeine, lithium, steroids, and adrenergic agonists), and by hereditary essential tremor. In *intention tremor,* the active limb oscillates more prominently as the limb approaches its target during goal-directed movements, though the tremor is present throughout the movement. **(p. 149)**

4.4 If a patient exhibits sudden jerks, sometimes simple, but sometimes as complex as well-organized voluntary movements, that persist in sleep, you would call these movements

A. Chorea.
B. Myoclonus.
C. Asterixis.
D. Tics.
E. Stereotypies.

The correct response is option D.

Tics are sudden jerks which can be simple or as complex as organized voluntary movements, such as touching an object or speaking a word. Tics differ from many other abnormal movements in that they may persist in sleep.

Chorea is characterized by irregular, rapid, flowing, nonstereotyped, and random involuntary movements. Myoclonus comprises sudden, jerky, shocklike movements that can originate at various levels in the nervous system. Asterixis is a momentary loss of postural tone that produces a flapping movement of the outstretched hand. Stereotypies are purposeless and repetitive movements that may be performed in lieu of other motor activity for long periods of time. **(pp. 150–151)**

4.5 In conducting a neurological examination of a patient, the examiner brings the reflex hammer toward the patient's mouth then to the side. What primitive reflex is being assessed?

A. Suck.
B. Rooting.
C. Snout.
D. Avoidance.
E. Nuchocephalic.

The correct response is option B.

Rooting is assessed by bringing an object, such as a reflex hammer, toward a patient's mouth and then to the side.

Sucking is assessed by inserting an object between the patient's lips; snouting by pressing on the patient's nasal philtrum. Avoidance is measured by stroking the patient's palm from proximal to distal or stroking the ulnar aspect of the patient's hand. The nuchocephalic reflex is assessed by briskly turning the shoulders of a standing patient whose eyes are closed. **(pp. 152, 153 [Table 4–3])**

4.6 Abulia may be defined as

A. The patient's continuing into present activity the elements of previous actions.
B. The patient's incapacity to carry out a sequential or ordered set of actions toward a unitary goal in the presence of the necessary objects.
C. The patient's lack of will, which in less severe form may include slowness, delayed response, laconic speech, and reduced initiative and effort.
D. The patient's incapacity to sustain activities that he or she was quite capable of beginning.
E. None of the above.

The correct response is option C.

Abulia or lack of will is a term used to describe loss of spontaneity due to cerebral disease.

Perseveration refers to the patient's continuing into present activity the elements of previous actions. Ideational apraxia is the incapacity to carry out a sequential or ordered set of actions toward a unitary goal in the presence of the necessary object. Impersistence is described as the incapacity of certain patients to sustain activities they were quite capable of beginning. **(pp. 164–166)**

4.7 A recently developed screening test, called the Frontal Assessment Battery, was developed by Dubois et al. (2000) primarily to assess

A. Executive cognitive dysfunction.
B. Dementia.
C. Focal cognitive syndromes.
D. HIV-related dementia.
E. Memory.

The correct response is option A.

Dubois et al. (2000) devised the Frontal Assessment Battery to identify executive dysfunction at the bedside. **(pp. 169 [Figure 4–3], 170)**

Reference

Dubois B, Slachevsky A, Litvan I, et al: The FAB: a Frontal Assessment Battery at bedside. Neurology 55:1621–1626, 2000

CHAPTER 5

Electrodiagnostic Techniques in Neuropsychiatry

Select the single best response for each question.

5.1 The electroencephalography (EEG) frequencies standard in clinical practice are reported in terms of particular ranges with corresponding Greek letters. All of the following ranges and referenced Greek-letter pairs are correct *except*

A. Gamma: >30 Hz.
B. Beta: 12–30 Hz.
C. Alpha: 8–12 Hz.
D. Theta: 4–7 Hz.
E. Delta: <1 Hz.

The correct response is option E.

Delta's range is 0.1–4.0 Hz.

The EEG frequency bands are defined as follows: gamma, >30 Hz; beta, 12–30 Hz; alpha, 8–12 Hz; theta, 4–7 Hz; and delta, 0.1–4.0 Hz. **(p. 191)**

5.2 Electroencephalography (EEG) has been used to establish electrophysiological correlates in panic disorder; indeed, because of its episodic nature, panic disorder is sometimes formulated as a seizure-like phenomenon. All of the following symptoms are common to simple partial seizures and panic attacks *except*

A. Fear.
B. Bradycardia.
C. Derealization.
D. Diaphoresis.
E. Abdominal discomfort.

The correct response is option B.

Tachycardia, not bradycardia, is a symptom of simple partial seizures and panic attacks. Fear, derealization, tachycardia, diaphoresis, and abdominal discomfort are characteristic symptoms of simple partial seizures with psychiatric and autonomic symptomatology. **(p. 193)**

5.3 Seizure activity and episodic aggression have been found to be clinically associated. As such, electroencephalography (EEG) may be useful clinically in evaluation of such patients. All of the following statements are true *except*

A. EEG abnormalities have been reported in approximately 50% of patients with antisocial personality disorder.
B. EEG abnormalities are more common in nonhabitual aggressors vs. habitual aggressors.
C. Bilateral paroxysmal EEG features are common in subjects who attack strangers.
D. An abnormal EEG may predict a favorable response to anticonvulsants in violent subjects.
E. Anticonvulsants may be beneficial in violent subjects even if the EEG is normal.

The correct response is option B.

Habitual aggressors have a fivefold increase in EEG abnormalities compared with nonhabitual aggressors.

Abnormal EEGs have been reported in 53% of patients diagnosed with antisocial personality disorder. Bilateral paroxysmal EEG features have been reported in 70% of subjects who have attacked strangers. The appearance of an abnormal EEG may predict a favorable therapeutic response to anticonvulsant medications. Studies have suggested that anticonvulsant therapy may have a beneficial effect on aggressive tendencies irrespective of the presence or absence of EEG abnormalities. **(p. 194)**

5.4 Electroencephalography (EEG) may be of use in the evaluation of cognitive disorders. Which of the following statements regarding the EEG in this group of illnesses is *true?*

A. A drop in background alpha of 1–2 Hz over a short period of time is not indicative of delirium as long as the alpha rhythm remains in the normal range.
B. Low-voltage beta activity increases in adults up to age 60 years and remains stable thereafter.
C. Mild diffuse slowing is pathological in individuals older than 75 years.
D. Focal delta activity in the anterior temporal areas is rare in patients older than 60 years.
E. EEG slowing is correlated with the severity of dementia and the number of senile plaques in Alzheimer's disease.

The correct response is option E.

EEG slowing has been found to be correlated with the severity of dementia and the number of senile plaques in Alzheimer's disease.

A drop of 1 Hz over a short period of time may be indicative of delirium, even though the alpha rhythm remains in the normal range. Low-voltage beta activity increases in adults up to age 60 years and declines thereafter. Mild diffuse slowing is found in approximately 20% of healthy individuals older than 75 years. Focal delta activity in the anterior temporal areas is seen in 30%–40% of patients older than 60 years. **(p. 195)**

5.5 Quantitative electroencephalography (QEEG) may have utility in the understanding of neuropsychiatric disorders and may even have prognostic significance. All of the following statements are true *except*

A. Schizophrenic patients have more delta activity compared with control subjects.
B. Delta activity is more pronounced in schizophrenic patients treated with antipsychotics.
C. Increased delta activity is present in children with high genetic loading for schizophrenia.
D. Alpha and beta power during photic stimulation is decreased in patients with presenile dementia.
E. Intoxication, delirium, and dementia are associated with increased delta activity.

The correct response is option B.

Delta activity is more pronounced in untreated schizophrenic patients.

Several studies have shown that schizophrenic patients have more delta activity, particularly over the frontal cortex, compared with control subjects. Increased delta activity is also present in children at genetic risk for schizophrenia and in cases of intoxication, delirium, and dementia. Alpha and beta power during photic stimulations is significantly decreased in patients with presenile dementia compared with age-matched controls. **(p. 197)**

5.6 Mild head injury is an oft-encountered problem in neuropsychiatric practice. Electroencephalography (EEG) may be helpful in evaluating these cases. Which of the following is *not* true of the EEG in head injury?

A. EEG has been shown to correlate with the admission Glasgow Coma Scale score for head injury.
B. Head injury features reduced theta activity.
C. Head injury features reduced beta activity.
D. Head injury features reduced alpha activity.
E. Frontal and temporal EEG abnormalities are common in mild head injury.

The correct response is option B.

Theta activity is increased in cases of mild head injury.

EEG at the time of hospital admission has been reported to correlate with Glasgow Coma Scale scores in patients with mild head injury. EEG changes that often accompany mild head injury are reduced beta and/or alpha activity and increased theta activity. Frontal lobe and temporal lobe EEG abnormalities are commonly reported in patients with mild head injury. **(p. 199)**

5.7 Pharmaco-electroencephalography (pharmaco-EEG) in clinical applications offers an attractive technique to fine-tune drug development, and is likely to play an expanded role in the future of applied psychopharmacology. All of the following statements are true *except*

A. Decreased quantitative electroencephalography (QEEG) theta and alpha activity have been reported in schizophrenic patients treated with high-potency antipsychotics.
B. Slow alpha changes identify nonresponders vs. responders to antipsychotics.
C. Medication-associated increases in beta waves correlate with decrease in depression symptoms.
D. QEEG profile after a single dose of an acetylcholinesterase inhibitor predicted cognitive modifications in dementia patients.
E. With antipsychotic treatment, increased QEEG alpha activity correlates with a favorable clinical response.

The correct response is option A.

An increase of QEEG theta and alpha activity, more often in the slow alpha range (7.5–9.5 Hz), has been reported in patients with schizophrenia treated with high-potency neuroleptics.

It has been found that slow alpha changes enable the identification of responders and nonresponders to antipsychotics with an overall accuracy ranging from 89.3% to 91.3%.

Drug-induced increase of beta waves was found to correlate with the decrease of depression psychopathological ratings.

QEEG profile after a single dose of an acetylcholinesterase inhibitor was found to be a good predictor of cognitive modifications in patients with Alzheimer's disease.

Increased QEEG alpha activity correlates with a favorable clinical response to antipsychotic treatment. **(p. 201)**

5.8 Evoked potentials, particularly the P300 potential, may be useful in the diagnosis and management of neuropsychiatric illness. All of the following statements are true *except*

A. The most consistent P300 finding in schizophrenia is a reduction in amplitude.
B. In schizophrenia, P300 abnormalities are present in nonmedicated and medicated patients.
C. P300 abnormalities correlate with the amount of negative symptoms and formal thought disorder in schizophrenia.
D. In schizophrenia, asymmetrical auditory P300 reduction is frequently reported, with smaller amplitudes over the right temporal region.
E. P300 abnormalities have been reported in relatives of schizophrenia patients and high-risk subjects for psychosis.

The correct response is option D.

Asymmetrical auditory P300 reduction in schizophrenia has been often reported with smaller amplitudes over the left temporal regions.

Several studies have found that schizophrenic patients have abnormal P300 potentials. P300 abnormalities are evident in both medicated and drug-free patients and are associated with several clinical features of schizophrenia, including negative symptoms, thought disorder, illness duration, and age at onset. P300 amplitude reduction or left-lateralized deficit has also been reported in first-degree relatives of schizophrenic patients, in high-risk subjects, and in psychosis-prone groups. **(pp. 202–203)**

CHAPTER 6

The Neuropsychological Evaluation

Select the single best response for each question.

6.1 Depressed patients without psychotic features often underperform, in comparison with control subjects, in all of the following functional areas *except*

A. Measures of speed of processing.
B. Mental flexibility.
C. Executive function.
D. Memory.
E. None of the above.

The correct response is option D.

Memory impairment is not a consistent finding in depressed patients without psychotic features, and memory performance may be intact even when memory complaints are present.

Depressed patients often underperform on measures of speed of processing, mental flexibility, and executive function compared with controls. Cognitive deficits, including memory, are more common in depressed patients with psychotic features than in depressed patients with no psychotic features. The degree of cognitive impairment appears to be related to the number of prior depressive episodes. **(pp. 218–219)**

6.2 One approach to neuropsychological testing is the use of a fixed battery of tests. Which of the following is an advantage of such an approach?

A. It allows the neuropsychologist to focus on a specific area of difficulty.
B. It enables the examiner to cover an area relevant for a diagnosis.
C. The patient receives a broad-based examination.
D. The examination usually will be brief, lasting only 1–2 hours.
E. All aspects of neuropsychological functioning will be examined.

The correct response is option C.

The advantage of fixed batteries is that the patient receives a fairly broad-based examination, which frequently lasts from 6 to 8 hours.

The fixed-battery approach does not focus on specific areas of difficulty for most patients, nor can it cover all areas relevant for either a reliable diagnosis or practical counseling. Moreover, aspects of neuropsychological functioning not included in a fixed battery will not be examined. **(p. 220)**

6.3 Patients may usually be grouped into one of the standard aphasia syndromes. Which of the following is *not* one of these syndromes?

A. Spontaneous aphasia.
B. Receptive aphasia.
C. Expressive aphasia.
D. Conduction aphasia.
E. Anomic aphasia.

The correct response is option A.

Spontaneous aphasia is not grouped with the other forms of aphasia.

Persons with aphasia tend to be grouped according to whether the main disorder is in language comprehension (receptive aphasia), expression (expressive aphasia), repetition (conduction aphasia), or naming (anomic aphasia). **(p. 226)**

6.4 Memory is a cognitive function frequently impaired by brain disorders. Which of the following statements regarding the neuropsychological effects of brain injury is *true*?

A. Left-hemispheric lesions are most likely to produce visuospatial memory impairments.
B. In most cases of brain injury, patients with memory impairment usually perform poorly on tests of fund of information or recall of remote events.
C. Most brain-injured patients will retain information learned before the injury as compared with new learning.
D. Right-hemispheric lesions are most likely to produce primarily verbal memory deficits.
E. Patients frequently will have anterograde amnesia without significant retrograde amnesia.

The correct response is option C.

Memory for information learned before brain injury is relatively preserved compared with new learning.

Left-hemisphere lesions are most likely to produce verbal memory deficits, whereas visuospatial memory impairments are associated with right-hemisphere lesions. Many patients with memory impairment perform relatively well on tests of fund of information or recall of remote events. In rare cases, patients will have retrograde amnesia without significant anterograde amnesia. **(p. 228)**

6.5 Executive functions include the ability to formulate a goal, to plan, to carry out goal-directed plans effectively, and to monitor and self-correct spontaneously and reliably. All of the following tests measure aspects of executive functioning *except*

A. The Tower of London.
B. Behavioral Assessment of the Dysexecutive Syndrome (BADS).
C. Twenty Questions test.
D. The Wisconsin Card Sorting Test (WCST).
E. The Complex Figure test.

The correct response is option E.

The Complex Figure test is a neuropsychological assessment that measures visuospatial processing, not executive functioning.

The Tower of London test assesses planning and foresight. The BADS is used to bring out problems with flexibility, planning, and priority setting in patients with brain injury and schizophrenia. The Twenty Questions test is used to judge priority-setting in tasks. The WCST measures adaptive decision making. All of these tests measure executive functioning. **(pp. 229, 230, 231 [Figure 6–5], 232)**

6.6 Which of the following tests is a self-report of symptoms associated with psychiatric disorders when they occur at high frequency levels?

A. The Hiscock and Hiscock Digit Memory Test.
B. The Symptom Checklist–90—Revised (SCL-90-R).
C. The Test of Memory Malingering (TOMM).
D. The Symptom Validity Test.
E. The Tinkertoy Test.

The correct response is option B.

The SCL-90-R (Derogatis 1983) is a self-report test of symptoms associated with psychiatric disorders when they occur at high frequency levels.

The Hiscock and Hiscock Digit Memory Test assesses the validity of memory complaints by requiring the patient to recall a short series of numbers using a forced-choice, two-item recognition task. The TOMM evaluates complaint validity by asking the patient to choose which pictures had been shown to him or her previously using a similar forced-choice technique. The Symptom Validity Test is used to diagnose people faking brain damage that tend to exaggerate poor performance on testing. The fundamental procedure examines the patient's complaints of inability by forcing a response to a simple, two-alternative problem involving the complaint. Using many trials, the examiner can calculate the likelihood that the performance deviates from chance or from expected performance. The Tinkertoy Test is a less structured test, in which the patient decides what to build and how to design it. Because there are few rules, the patient's level of productivity on this task typically reflects his or her level of productivity in the real world. **(pp. 232–233)**

Reference

Derogatis LR: Symptom Checklist 90–Revised (SCL-90-R). Towson, MD, Clinical Psychometric Research, 1983

CHAPTER 7

Clinical and Functional Imaging in Neuropsychiatry

Select the single best response for each question.

7.1 Neuroimaging has revolutionized the clinical practice of neuropsychiatry. For many psychiatric conditions, information obtained from brain imaging studies may assist with differential diagnosis, suggest a treatment plan, and inform prognosis. Which of the following conditions would *not* be considered an indication for neuroimaging?

A. Poison/toxin exposure.
B. Traumatic brain injury.
C. Dementia.
D. Catatonia.
E. Relapse of established psychotic illness.

The correct response is option E.

Neuroimaging would not be indicated in the relapse of an established psychotic illness.

Clinical indications for neuroimaging include poison/toxin exposure, traumatic brain injury, significant alcohol abuse, seizure disorders with psychiatric symptoms, movement disorders, autoimmune disorders, eating disorders, and delirium. Clinical signs or symptoms warranting brain imaging studies include dementia or cognitive decline, new onset of mental illness after age 50 years, initial psychotic break, presentation at an atypical age for diagnosis, focal neurological signs, catatonia, and sudden personality changes. **(p. 246, Table 7–2)**

7.2 Noncontrast computed tomography (CT) of the brain remains the standard neuroimaging in neuropsychiatric practice for many conditions. Which of the following tissue types has a characteristic white appearance in noncontrast CT scans?

A. Water.
B. Cerebrospinal fluid.
C. Gray matter.
D. Clotted blood.
E. White matter.

The correct response is option D.

Clotted blood, bone, and calcified tissue appear white in a noncontrast CT scan.

Water and cerebrospinal fluid appear nearly black, gray matter appears light gray, and white matter appears medium gray. **(p. 249, Table 7–3)**

7.3 In magnetic resonance imaging (MRI), spin echo pulse sequences include T1-weighted, T2-weighted, and fluid-attenuated inversion recovery (FLAIR) sequences. Generally, the T2 and FLAIR sequences are superior for the interpretation of neuropathology. Which of the following tissues appears differently in T2-weighted vs. FLAIR images?

A. Cerebrospinal fluid.
B. Bone.
C. Gray matter.
D. White matter.
E. Blood.

The correct response is option A.

Cerebrospinal fluid appears white in T2-weighted images and black in FLAIR images.

Bone and blood appear black in both images, gray matter appears medium gray, and white matter appears dark gray. **(pp. 255–256, Table 7–4)**

7.4 The neuropsychiatrist must frequently choose the most clinically appropriate neuroimaging modality for the case at hand. Which of the following clinical conditions is preferentially imaged with computed tomography (CT), as opposed to magnetic resonance imaging (MRI)?

A. Subcortical lesions.
B. Poison/toxin exposure.
C. Acute hemorrhage.
D. Eating disorders.
E. Demyelinating disease.

The correct response is option C.

Acute hemorrhage, calcified lesions, and bone injury are preferentially imaged with CT. Subcortical lesions, poison/toxin exposure, eating disorders, and demyelinating disorders are preferentially imaged with MRI. **(p. 260 [Table 7–5])**

7.5 Positron emission tomography (PET) and single-photon emission computed tomography (SPECT) offer a more dynamic assessment of neuropsychiatric illnesses because of their sensitivity to neural function, not just anatomical structure. Which of the following neuronal functions can be assessed with PET but not with SPECT?

A. Glucose uptake (regional cerebral metabolic rate [rCMR]).
B. Blood flow (regional cerebral blood flow [rCBF]).
C. Serotonin transporter binding.
D. Serotonin receptor binding.
E. Acetylcholine nicotinic receptor binding.

The correct response is option A.

Glucose uptake cannot be assessed with SPECT. All of the other functions listed can be assessed with both PET and SPECT. **(p. 264 [Table 7–6])**

7.6 In the clinical application of positron emission tomography (PET) and single-photon emission computed tomography (SPECT), technical and logistical considerations may make one method preferable to the other. Which of the following statements is *false*?

A. PET has higher spatial resolution than SPECT.
B. PET nearly eliminates attenuation artifacts.
C. SPECT is more widely available and less expensive than PET.
D. Reimbursement for PET is limited to its use for differentiating between Alzheimer's disease and Lewy body dementia.
E. On-site cyclotrons are no longer typically needed for PET scanners.

The correct response is option D.

Reimbursement for PET is currently limited to distinguishing frontotemporal dementia from Alzheimer's disease, presurgical evaluation of intractable epilepsy, and distinguishing radiation necrosis from recurrent brain tumors.

PET has the advantages of higher spatial resolution and true attenuation correction, nearly eliminating attenuation artifacts. SPECT has the advantage of being more widely available, less expensive, and reimbursable for most conditions. The old requirement of on-site cyclotrons has been obviated by the establishment of numerous commercial cyclotrons throughout the country. **(pp. 268, 270)**

7.7 One of the most useful applications of functional imaging is in the evaluation of dementia, where functional imaging may assist in elucidating the type of dementia to guide early treatment. All of the following statements are true *except*

A. Alzheimer's disease features bilateral posterior temporoparietal decreased perfusion/metabolism.
B. With progression of Alzheimer's disease, frontal lobes also exhibit decreased perfusion/metabolism.
C. In Alzheimer's disease, occipital cortex is usually preserved.
D. Positron emission tomography (PET)/single-photon emission computed tomography (SPECT) of Parkinson's dementia can be clearly distinguished from SPECT/PET of Alzheimer's disease.
E. SPECT/PET can readily differentiate Alzheimer's disease from frontotemporal dementia (FTD).

The correct response is option D.

Parkinson's patients often develop dementia but the SPECT/PET appearance has not been characterized and likely overlaps with both Alzheimer's disease and Lewy body dementia.

Approximately one-third of patients with Alzheimer's disease exhibit bilateral, symmetrical posterior temporoparietal decreased perfusion or metabolism. Frequently, the abnormalities are asymmetrical and may initially involve only the temporal or parietal cortex. As the disease progresses, the frontal and occasionally the occipital lobes become involved with decreased perfusion. SPECT/PET scanning demonstrates reduced perfusion of the frontal and/or anterior temporal cortex in frontotemporal dementia (e.g., Pick's disease), which is usually readily distinguished from Alzheimer's disease and Lewy body dementia. **(pp. 270–271)**

7.8 Regarding the use of single-photon emission computed tomography (SPECT)/positron emission tomography (PET) studies in vascular disease, which of the following statements is *true*?

A. Small vessel disease (e.g., Binswanger's disease) has a highly specific SPECT/PET appearance.
B. In acute stroke, SPECT is preferred to CT, because CT is insufficiently accurate in identifying hemorrhagic stroke.
C. Compromised vascular reserve, which may be normal on baseline SPECT, may be visualized following intravenous injection of acetazolamide.
D. Arterioles distal to an obstruction dilate robustly following intravenous injection of acetazolamide.
E. Multi-infarct dementia features multiple moderate-sized defects with diffuse boundaries.

The correct response is option C.

Compromised vascular reserve can be visualized on a SPECT scan performed following intravenous injection of acetazolamide.

Small vessel disease (e.g., Binswanger's disease) is *not* associated with a specific SPECT/PET pattern. In acute stroke, computed tomography (CT) scanning can be obtained more quickly than SPECT or PET and is quite accurate. Arterioles distal to an arterial obstruction cannot dilate further in response to acetazolamide. SPECT/PET reveals defects with well-defined boundaries in multi-infarct dementia. **(p. 274)**

CHAPTER 8

Epidemiological and Genetic Aspects of Neuropsychiatric Disorders

Select the single best response for each question.

8.1 The probability that an individual will develop a disease over a specified time is known as

A. Prevalence.
B. Incidence.
C. Rate.
D. Risk.
E. None of the above.

The correct response is option D.

Risk refers to the probability that an individual will develop a disease over a specified time.

Prevalence is the number of existing cases of a disease at a given point in time as a proportion of the total population. *Incidence* is the number of new cases of a disease during a given period as a proportion of the total population at risk. *Rate* is the measure of individuals newly developing a disease in relation to the subject number that remain at risk. **(p. 302)**

8.2 A number of research strategies have been developed to elucidate genetic and epidemiological aspects of neuropsychiatric disorders. Which of the following is used to determine the genetic contribution to a disorder?

A. Family studies.
B. Twin studies.
C. High-risk studies.
D. Segregation analysis.
E. Linkage analysis.

The correct response is option B.

Twin studies are used to resolve the genetic contribution to a disorder.

Family studies are used to examine the risk in which patterns of disease are distributed within families. In *high-risk studies,* individuals who are at risk for a disorder are followed up prospectively. *Segregation analysis* tests explicit models about the inheritance of disease genes on existing family data by comparing the distribution of illness observed in family members with that predicted by a given genetic hypothesis. *Linkage analysis* is a strategy for isolating a gene of unknown structure or function based on its chromosomal location. **(pp. 303–304)**

8.3 Which of the following statements concerning single-nucleotide polymorphisms (SNPs) is *false*?

A. SNPs are DNA sequence variations.
B. SNPs occur when a single nucleotide (A, T, C, or G) in the genome sequence is altered.
C. SNPs can be in noncoding regions.
D. SNPs can be in genes that affect disease susceptibility.
E. SNPs result from a mutation in a restriction enzyme site.

The correct response is option E.

It is restriction fragment length polymorphisms (RFLPs), not SNPs, that result from a mutation in a restriction enzyme site.

SNPs are DNA sequence variations that occur when a single nucleotide (A, T, C, or G) in the genome sequence is altered. SNPs can be in noncoding regions or in genes that affect disease susceptibility or drug response, and they are becoming the marker of choice for genetic studies, since they are the most common form of variation in the human genome. **(pp. 305–306)**

8.4 All of the following statements concerning the genetics of Huntington's disease (HD) are true *except*

A. It is transmitted in an autosomal dominant fashion.
B. The gene responsible for HD was mapped to the short arm of chromosome 4.
C. Heterozygous inactivation of the HD gene as a result of chromosomal translocation is associated with an abnormal phenotype.
D. The genetic abnormality responsible for HD was identified as a CAG trinucleotide-repeat expansion in the first exon of a novel gene.
E. Age at onset of HD was found to be inversely related to the length of trinucleotide repeats in the gene.

The correct response is option C.

Heterozygous inactivation of the Huntington's disease gene is not associated with an abnormal phenotype.

HD is transmitted in an autosomal dominant fashion. In 1983, the gene responsible for HD was mapped to the short arm of chromosome 4 by the use of a linked polymorphic marker. Ten years later, the genetic abnormality for HD was identified as a CAG trinucleotide-repeat expansion in the first exon of a novel gene. Age at onset has been found to be inversely related to the length of trinucleotide repeats in the gene. **(p. 310)**

8.5 Which of the following statements about epidemiological findings in Parkinson's disease (PD) is *true*?

A. PD affects about 1% of adults older than 60 years.
B. The prevalence estimate of PD is 900 in 100,000.
C. The average age at onset of PD is 70 years but may be decreasing.
D. PD affects men and women equally.
E. Early-onset PD accounts for 2%–3% of patients.

The correct response is option A.

Parkinson's disease affects about 1% of adults older than 60 years.

The prevalence of PD is estimated at 133 in 100,000. The average age at onset is 63 years but may be increasing. PD may affect men at a slightly higher rate than women. Early-onset PD occurs between the ages of 21 and 40 years and accounts for 5%–10% of patients. **(pp. 313–314)**

8.6 Epidemiological findings concerning autism include all of the following *except*

A. Onset typically occurs before age 3 years.
B. The overall rate of autism in second-degree relatives of children with autism is 0.2%.
C. The male-to-female ratio is 1.5 to 1.0.
D. Rates of autism in siblings of affected individuals are in the range of 2%–6%.
E. The concordance rate for monozygotic twins has been estimated to be between 36% and 91%.

The correct response is option C.

A consistently observed male-to-female ratio of 3–4 to 1 has been noted, with females often having more severe impairment, particularly in IQ.

Onset of autism typically occurs before age 3 years. Several studies have suggested an overall rate of autism of 0.2% in second-degree relatives, 0.1% in third-degree relatives, and 2%–6% in siblings of affected individuals. The concordance rate has been estimated to be between 36% and 91% for monozygotic twins and between 0% and 24% for dizygotic twins. **(p. 318)**

8.7 Which of the following factors is associated with a lower risk of developing Alzheimer's disease (AD)?

A. Traumatic brain injury (TBI).
B. Chronic inflammation.
C. Female sex.
D. Cigarette smoking.
E. Higher educational level.

The correct response is option E.

A higher education level is a protective factor against AD, perhaps due to increased synaptic and/or dendritic complexity attendant to learning demands. Low educational attainment has been associated with a doubling of AD incidence.

Traumatic brain injury has been related to AD risk. A prospective study showed that TBI increased the incidence of AD by fourfold over the subsequent 5 years. There is strong support of a role for chronic inflammation in initiating and worsening AD. Use of nonsteroidal anti-inflammatory drugs (NSAIDs) has shown protective effects. Females have a greater risk for AD, even accounting for their longer lifespan, with males showing a higher rate of vascular dementia. It has been hypothesized that the risk for women could be due to menopause and many long-term studies suggested that women who take estrogen-based hormone replacement therapy (HRT) had a lower risk of developing AD. Cigarette smoking has been shown to increase AD risk, especially in men. **(p. 323)**

8.8 Family studies of bipolar disorder have demonstrated all of the following findings *except*

A. A sevenfold increase in lifetime risk for bipolar disorder in families with the disorder compared with family members of control subjects.
B. Recurrence risks were found to be higher in females, either of the relative or of the bipolar proband.
C. The age at onset of the first manic or depressive episode has been shown to be earlier in the younger generation of two generations of affected relative pairs.
D. The risk for bipolar disorder appears to be especially elevated in the relatives of probands with early-onset disorder.
E. The risk for bipolar disorder increases with the number of psychiatrically ill relatives.

The correct response is option B.

Recurrence risks do not vary by gender (either of the relative or of the bipolar proband).

A sevenfold increase in lifetime risk for bipolar disorder has been found in families of individuals with the disorder compared with families of control subjects. The age at onset of the first manic or depressive episode has been shown to be earlier, and the frequency of episodes greater, in the younger generation of two generations of affected relative pairs. **(p. 327)**

8.9 High-risk studies of obsessive-compulsive disorder (OCD) in children and adolescents have revealed which of the following?

A. Children with Sydenham's chorea show higher rates of OCD symptoms.
B. Females with early-onset OCD have persistent and severe symptoms.
C. Females with early-onset OCD have a higher incidence of birth complications than males.
D. Early-onset OCD predicts a lower rate of Tourette's disorder and tics in relatives.
E. After exclusion of Tourette's disorder from OCD probands, tics are not found to be more prevalent in OCD families.

The correct response is option A.

Studies of children with Sydenham's chorea, a neurological manifestation of rheumatic fever, led to the discovery that many children with this syndrome showed higher rates of obsessive-compulsive symptoms.

Males with early-onset OCD have been reported to have persistent and severe symptoms, as well as a higher incidence of birth complications than females, suggesting that males may be more vulnerable than females to the central nervous system damage that results in OCD. OCD co-occurs with tics and Tourette's disorder, particularly in males and individuals with early-onset OCD. Even when subjects with Tourette's disorder are excluded from the OCD cohort, studies still find tics to be more prevalent in OCD families. **(pp. 335–336)**

8.10 A 22-year-old female patient whom you are treating is concerned that she may develop schizophrenia, given that her mother has been treated for many years for paranoid schizophrenia. She asks you about her risk for developing the illness. The patient is an only child, and her biological father has no psychiatric history. This patient's risk rate is

A. 6%.
B. 13%.
C. 25%.
D. 46%.
E. 53%.

The correct response is option B.

First-degree relatives of schizophrenic probands have a risk rate of 13% when one parent is affected, 46% when both are. **(p. 338)**

CHAPTER 9

Neuropsychiatric Aspects of Pain Management

Select the single best response for each question.

9.1 Pain is processed by a series of neural tissues that are classified as providing ascending modulation, central processing, or descending inhibition. Which of the following structures is *not* involved in central processing?

A. Spinothalamic tracts.
B. Anterior cingulate gyrus.
C. Insular cortex.
D. Prefrontal cortex.
E. Somatosensory cortex.

The correct response is option A.

Central processing does not involve the spinothalamic tracts.

Cortical or central processing involves several key areas: the anterior cingulate gyrus and the insular, prefrontal, inferior parietal, primary and secondary somatosensory, primary motor, and premotor cortices. **(pp. 366–367)**

9.2 Within central processing, the "medial" system is responsible for generating the affective/emotional component of pain, while the "lateral" system is responsible for the discriminative sensory components. Which of the following structures is part of the medial system?

A. Primary somatosensory cortex (SI).
B. Secondary somatosensory cortex (SII).
C. Anterior cingulate.
D. Parietal cortex.
E. Premotor cortex.

The correct response is option C.

The anterior cingulate and the insular cortex are thought to be a part of the "medial pain system," responsible for generating the affective/emotional component of pain.

The somatosensory cortex (SI and SII) and the parietal cortex have been postulated as forming part of the "lateral" pain system, which is thought to be involved in the discriminative sensory components of pain. **(p. 367)**

9.3 The relationship between pain and mood disorders is of great clinical relevance to neuropsychiatrists, who frequently treat patients with these comorbid conditions. All of the following statements are true *except*

A. Patients with pain score higher on measures of depression than do patients without pain.
B. In cancer patients, depressive symptoms are more highly correlated with pain than with a history of previous clinical depression.
C. Depression is the most common psychiatric diagnosis among chronic pain patients.
D. The presence or absence of mood symptoms has a differential effect on the opioid responsiveness of pain.
E. Emotional aspects of pain, such as depression, are modulated by the insular cortex.

The correct response is option E.

Emotional aspects of pain are mediated by the anterior cingulate gyrus in conjunction with amygdala and limbic structures, whereas sensory aspects are controlled by the parietal and insular cortices.

Patients with pain score higher on measures of depression, anxiety, and other signs of mood disturbance than those with little or no pain. The presence of significant pain among cancer patients is more strongly associated with major depressive symptoms than is a prior life history of depression. Depression is the most frequently reported psychiatric diagnosis among chronic pain patients. In a study conducted by Wasan et al. in 2004, 48% of patients with a low level of psychiatric symptoms had a good response to opioid analgesia, while only 20% of patients with a high level of psychiatric symptoms experienced relief. **(pp. 368–369)**

9.4 Many chemicals present in blood and tissue are algesic. Which of the following substances does *not* itself directly excite primary noxious afferents?

A. Prostaglandins.
B. Serotonin.
C. Histamine.
D. Acetylcholine.
E. Bradykinin.

The correct response is option A.

Prostaglandins do not excite pain fibers; however, they appear to sensitize primary afferents to painful substances.

Serotonin, histamine, acetylcholine, bradykinin, slow-reacting substance of anaphylaxis (SRS-A), calcitonin gene–related peptide (CGRP), and potassium all excite primary noxious afferents. **(p. 370)**

9.5 The dorsal horn of the spinal cord is divided into different laminae, each with specific roles in neural transmission. Which of these laminae is also known as the substantia gelatinosa and is the site of spinal cord opiate analgesia?

A. Lamina I.
B. Lamina II.
C. Lamina III.
D. Lamina IV.
E. Lamina X.

The correct response is option B.

Lamina II is also known as "substantia gelatinosa." The clinical phenomenon of selective spinal cord opiate analgesia is mediated through opioid receptors found in lamina II.

The dorsal horn of the spinal cord is organized into distinct laminae, with specific primary afferent terminals found in individual laminae. **(pp. 372–373)**

9.6 Which of the following laminae does not contribute axons to the spinothalamic tract?

A. Lamina I.
B. Lamina IV.
C. Lamina V.
D. Lamina VII.
E. Lamina X.

The correct response is option E.

Lamina X does not contribute axons that make up the spinothalamic tract.

Axons from laminae I, IV, V, VII, and VIII make up the spinothalamic tract. These axons ascend predominantly in the contralateral ventral quadrant of the spinal cord. Crossed fibers predominate, but neuroanatomical studies have indicated that perhaps 25% of all fibers ascend in the ipsilateral ventral quadrant. These spinothalamic fibers subsequently ascend to the thalamus. **(p. 374)**

9.7 Which of the following analgesics is not a cyclooxygenase inhibitor?

A. Acetaminophen.
B. Aspirin.
C. Indomethacin.
D. Diclofenac.
E. Keterolac.

The correct response is option A.

Acetaminophen is not a cyclooxygenase inhibitor.

Aspirin, indomethacin, ibuprofen, diclofenac, and keterolac are all cyclooxygenase inhibitors. **(pp. 377, 380–381)**

9.8 Treatment of pain states may be an appropriate application of tricyclic antidepressants (TCAs). Unfortunately, a host of cardiac concerns make electrocardiogram (ECG) monitoring necessary with these agents. Which of the following is *not* a characteristic ECG change associated with TCAs?

A. Flattened T-wave.
B. Prolonged Q-T interval.
C. Prolonged QRS interval.
D. Prolonged PR interval.
E. Elevated S-T segment.

The correct response is option E.

Elevated S-T segments are not an ECG change associated with TCAs.

ECG changes observed with TCA use include flattened T-waves; prolonged Q-T, QRS, and PR intervals; and depressed S-T segments. **(p. 384)**

9.9 Anticonvulsants are an often helpful class of medications for neuropathic pain. Unfortunately, they are well known to be associated with a series of side effects that may limit their use. Which of the following agents is associated with cognitive slowing and renal stones?

A. Topiramate.
B. Carbamazepine.
C. Levetiracetam.
D. Gabapentin.
E. Lamotrigine.

The correct response is option A.

Reported side effects of topiramate include kidney stones and cognitive slowing, in addition to somnolence, dizziness, ataxia, paresthesias, nervousness, abnormal vision, and weight loss.

Side effects of carbamazepine include sedation, nausea, diplopia, vertigo, hematological abnormalities, jaundice, oliguria, hypertension, and acute left ventricular heart failure. The side effects of levetiracetam include somnolence, asthenia, dizziness, depression, and nervousness. Side effects of gabapentin include somnolence, dizziness, ataxia, fatigue, concentration difficulties, gastrointestinal disturbance, nystagmus, and pedal edema. Lamotrigine's side effects include dizziness, nausea, headache, ataxia, diplopia, blurred vision, somnolence, and Stevens-Johnson syndrome. **(p. 385 [Table 9–5])**

Reference

Wasan A, Davar G, Jamison R, et al: Psychiatric comorbidity diminishes opioid analgesia in patients with discogenic low back pain (abstract no 845). J Pain 5 (suppl 1):S70, 2004

CHAPTER 10

Neuropsychiatric Aspects of Disorders of Attention

Select the single best response for each question.

10.1 "An alert state in which individuals are aware of self and environment" is a definition of

A. Attentional capacity.
B. Consciousness.
C. Selective attention.
D. Response selection and executive control.
E. Sustained attention.

The correct response is option B.

Consciousness is an alert state in which individuals are "aware of self and environment."

Humans have a limited capacity for attention. *Attentional capacity* governs both the amount of information that can be handled and the intensity of cognitive processing that can be performed on that information. Processes that enable or facilitate the selection of salient information for further cognitive processing are collectively referred to as *selective attention*. A wide variety of processes are associated with *response selection and executive control*, ranging from simple behavioral orienting to more complex cognitive processes involving intention, planning, and decision making. *Sustained attention* depends on the cyclical reprocessing of information that provides positive and negative feedback from the results of prior actions. **(pp. 406, 408, 409)**

10.2 A number of different brain regions are involved in attentional processes. Which brain region plays a pivotal role in attention by contributing important energetic components of drive and motivation?

A. Dorsolateral prefrontal cortex.
B. Reticular activating system (RAS).
C. Hypothalamus.
D. Anterior cingulate gyrus.
E. Orbitomedial prefrontal circuit.

The correct response is option D.

The anterior cingulate gyrus plays a pivotal role in attention by contributing important energetic components of drive and motivation.

The dorsolateral prefrontal cortex is involved in maintaining response flexibility and generating response alternatives, working memory, and the temporal sequencing of information. The RAS plays a major role in modulating arousal and provides global regulation of attentional tone for the forebrain. The hypothalamus influences the intensity of arousal and the direction of attention. The orbitomedial prefrontal circuit modulates impulses and participates in the regulation of mood and working memory. **(pp. 410, 411, 412)**

10.3 A number of tasks place demands on attentional capacity and focus because of the requirement to divide attention or to inhibit interfering stimuli or responses. An example is a test in which the subject is required to name the color of a word while ignoring the actual word. What is the name of this test?

A. Wisconsin Card Sorting Test.
B. Trail Making Test.
C. Controlled Word Association Test.
D. Continuous Performance Test.
E. Stroop Test.

The correct response is option E.

In the Stroop Test, the subject is required to name the color of a word while ignoring the actual word. Interference is created because the color and the meaning of the word are mismatched. This test places strong demands on inhibitory systems, which must suppress both the other stimulus feature and a strong response tendency.

The Wisconsin Card Sorting Test measures concept formation and hypothesis testing. Subjects are presented with cards containing features for color, shape, and number. The task is to determine the correct category for a response based on feedback provided by the examiner. Subjects sort cards to the appropriate category but must switch to a new category when the response criteria change. Poor performance on the WCST is often associated with impairments of conceptual flexibility and switching and perseveration secondary to frontal lobe damage affecting the dorsolateral region.

With the Trail Making Test, subjects are initially required to connect a sequence of numbers by drawing a line between numbers that are placed randomly on a sheet of paper (Trails A). On Trails B, subjects are required to alternate between numbers and letters in ascending order. Errors occur when the patient fails to alternate and connects two letters or numbers or when there is a break in the sequence and a particular item is omitted. Each task is timed.

In the Controlled Word Association Test, subjects are given 60 seconds to produce as many words as possible that start with a particular letter (F, A, or S) or that belong to a specific semantic category (animals). The total number of words generated is then scored.

The Continuous Performance Test measures signal detection performance over blocks of trials. Visual or auditory stimuli are presented sequentially. Intermixed among distractor stimuli are particular target stimuli, such as the letter *A*. The task is to respond to the target and not to the distractors. **(pp. 417, 419, 420)**

10.4 A number of psychophysiological and neuroimaging techniques have been used to assess the neurobiological substrates of attention. A test that measures the random thermal motion of water in brain tissue has been used to examine brain dysfunction in a clinical population. What is this test called?

A. Event-related potential (ERP).
B. Functional magnetic resonance imaging (fMRI).
C. Diffusion tensor imaging (DTI).
D. Electroencephalogram (EEG).
E. Autonomic studies.

The correct response is option C.

DTI measures the random thermal motion of water in brain tissue.

ERP consists of a series of specific positive and negative voltage deflections, used to measure brain responses that are the direct result of a thought or perception. Functional magnetic resonance imaging is used to examine human brain function associated with neuroscientific constructs such as attention. fMRI yields better spatial resolution than positron emission tomography (PET) or ERP. EEG is the neurophysiological measurement of electrical activity of the brain. EEGs are most useful in the diagnosis of epilepsy and syncope, sleep disorders, eating disorders, coma, and brain death. Autonomic studies use skin conductance response and cardiovascular measures, such as changes in heart rate. Autonomic measures reflect task-specific attentional activation. **(pp. 421, 422, 423)**

10.5 Neglect and deficits in attention are important clinical findings in patients with neuropsychiatric disorders. Which of the following statements concerning these impairments is *false*?

A. Neglect usually occurs relative to the right side of space, which illustrates the importance of the dominant hemisphere in spatial attention.
B. Hemi-inattention and neglect are manifestations of unilateral brain lesions.
C. Lesions affecting the reticular system that produce neglect also involve significant arousal and activation impairments.
D. Unilateral basal ganglia damage often results in impairments of both hemi-attention and intention.
E. Cingulate lesions are more likely to affect intention than sensory selective attention.

The correct response is option A.

Neglect usually occurs relative to the *left* side of space, which illustrates the importance of the nondominant hemisphere in spatial attention.

Hemi-inattention and neglect are manifestations of unilateral brain lesions. Striking spatial asymmetry in attentional performance is a central feature of these syndromes. Lesions affecting the reticular system that produce neglect also involve significant arousal and activation impairments. Unilateral basal ganglia damage often results in impairments of hemi-attention and intention, reflecting the importance of this system to sensorimotor integration. Cingulate lesions are more likely to affect intention than sensory selective attention. **(p. 426)**

10.6 Which of the following statements concerning attention-deficit/hyperactivity disorder (ADHD) is *false*?

A. For the most part, patients with ADHD have normal intelligence.
B. In ADHD, the attention deficit results from susceptibility to distraction.
C. Impaired sustained attention is a primary feature of ADHD.
D. Children with ADHD exhibit more errors of both omission and commission on the Continuous Performance Test than do children without ADHD.
E. Patients with ADHD do not exhibit major cognitive dysfunction.

The correct response is option B.

On laboratory tests, children with ADHD rarely show problems with performance in the presence of distracting information. Thus, attentional filtering may not be the major problem in most cases of ADHD.

For the most part, patients with ADHD have normal intelligence and do not exhibit major cognitive dysfunction. Impaired sustained attention is a primary feature of ADHD. Impairments are greatest when vigilance is required to detect infrequent information, particularly when this information is not motivationally salient. Hyperactive children exhibit more errors of both omission and commission on the Continuous Performance Test than do children without ADHD, and they also show more rapid deterioration of task performance over time. **(p. 432)**

CHAPTER 11

Neuropsychiatric Aspects of Delirium

Select the single best response for each question.

11.1 The diagnostic criteria for delirium as reflected in the DSM series have evolved significantly over time. Which version first specifically included dysexecutive symptoms in the criteria for delirium?

A. DSM-I (American Psychiatric Association 1952).
B. DSM-II (American Psychiatric Association 1968).
C. DSM-III-R (American Psychiatric Association 1987).
D. DSM-IV (American Psychiatric Association 1994).
E. None of the above.

The correct response is option E.

Dysexecutive symptoms (i.e., impairment of prefrontal executive cognition) are not mentioned in any DSM edition, despite the importance of prefrontal involvement in delirium. **(p. 447)**

11.2 Misdiagnosis of delirium, a common clinical problem, has been found to be more likely among certain patient populations. Which of the following clinical attributes is *not* a risk factor for such misdiagnosis?

A. Hyperactive patient presentation.
B. Advanced patient age.
C. Sensory impairments.
D. Preexisting dementia.
E. Intensive care setting.

The correct response is option A.

Hyperactive presentation is not typical of delirium.

Misdiagnosis of delirium is more likely among patients who are older; who have sensory impairments, preexisting dementia, or a hypoactive presentation; and who are referred from surgical or intensive care settings. Delirium is commonly misdiagnosed as depression by nonpsychiatrists. **(p. 449)**

11.3 The distinction between delirium and dementia is rendered problematic by several overlapping symptoms that are common to these two cognitive disorders. Which dementia syndrome, characterized by fluctuating symptom severity, visual hallucinations, attentional impairment, altered state of consciousness, and delusions, is particularly difficult to distinguish from delirium?

A. Dementia due to hypothyroidism.
B. Dementia due to HIV disease.
C. Alzheimer's dementia.
D. Vascular dementia.
E. Lewy body dementia.

The correct response is option E.

Lewy body dementia mimics delirium in its characteristic fluctuations in symptoms over time. **(pp. 449–450, 498)**

11.4 In their study examining differences in symptom profile between patients with delirium and patients with dementia, which of the following symptoms were found by Trzepacz et al. (2002) to be more common in delirium than in dementia?

A. Delusions.
B. Affective lability.
C. Thought process abnormalities.
D. Disorders of short-term memory.
E. Disorders of long-term memory.

The correct response is option C.

Trzepacz et al. (2002) noted significant differences between delirium and dementia for thought process abnormalities, sleep-wake cycle disturbances, motor agitation, attention, and visuospatial ability, which were more impaired in delirium.

No differences between the disorders were found for delusions, affective lability, language, motor retardation, orientation, and short- or long-term memory. **(p. 450)**

11.5 Delirium following stroke is unfortunately a common clinical scenario for the neuropsychiatrist. Which of the following statements regarding the relationship between delirium and stroke is *false?*

A. Delirium complicates the course of acute stroke in nearly 50% of patients.
B. Delirium more commonly follows ischemic than hemorrhagic stroke.
C. Anticholinergic medications carry a particularly high risk of delirium in stroke patients.
D. Poststroke delirium is more common with hemispheric stroke than with brain stem stroke.
E. Delirium is more common following intracerebral rather than subarachnoid hemorrhage or infarct.

The correct response is option B.

Delirium is more common after hemorrhagic, rather than ischemic, stroke.

Delirium can complicate the acute course of stroke in up to 48% of patients. Anticholinergic medications pose a particular risk of causing delirium in stroke patients. Delirium is more common after hemispherical than brain stem or cerebellar stroke—in particular, right middle cerebral artery lesions—and after intracerebral rather than subarachnoid hemorrhage or cerebral infarct. **(pp. 464–465)**

11.6 The distinction between "core" and "associated" delirium symptoms may be helpful in understanding delirium phenomenology. Which of the following is considered a "core" symptom of delirium?

A. Illusions.
B. Hallucinations.
C. Delusions.
D. Affective changes.
E. Language disturbances.

The correct response is option E.

Language disturbances, together with attentional deficits, memory impairments, disorientation, sleep-wake cycle disturbance, thought process abnormalities, and motoric alterations, are considered "core" symptoms of delirium.

"Associated" or noncore symptoms include perceptual disturbances, such as illusions and hallucinations, delusions, and affective changes. **(p. 477)**

11.7 Which of the following atypical antipsychotics, by virtue of its multiple receptor effects (including sedation, anticholinergic properties, and lowering of the seizure threshold), should not be used in delirium?

A. Risperidone.
B. Ziprasidone.
C. Aripiprazole.
D. Clozapine.
E. Olanzapine.

The correct response is option D.

Clozapine, the first atypical antipsychotic, is clinically distinct from the others and is not recommended for treatment of delirium, because it is very sedating, has significant anticholinergic side effects, causes sinus tachycardia, lowers the seizure threshold, and is associated with causing agranulocytosis. Clozapine-induced delirium can be reversed with cholinergic agents. **(p. 491)**

11.8 A final common neural pathway for delirium would encompass both neuroanatomical and neurochemical dimensions. The preponderance of evidence in the literature supports which of the following as the likely final common neural pathway in delirium?

A. Low cholinergic/high dopaminergic state.
B. High cholinergic/high dopaminergic state.
C. High γ-aminobutyric acid (GABA)/low dopaminergic state.
D. Low GABA/high dopaminergic state.
E. Low serotonin/high GABA state.

The correct response is option A.

A low cholinergic/high dopaminergic state is the proposed final common neural pathway for delirium.

Although other neurotransmitter systems are known to be involved for certain etiologies (e.g., hepatic insufficiency or alcohol withdrawal deliria), the activity of cholinergic and dopaminergic pathways can be regulated and affected by other neurotransmitters, including serotonergic, opiatergic, GABAergic, noradrenergic, and glutamatergic systems; altered metabolic states; physiological changes of inflammatory and stress responses; and glial activity. Thus, many factors can interact with the final common pathway to culminate in delirium. **(p. 495)**

11.9 Electroencephalography (EEG) may be a helpful diagnostic tool in clarifying cases of delirium, particularly in regard to differential causes of delirium. An EEG pattern of "low-voltage fast activity" is consistent with which of the following delirium etiologies?

A. Anticholinergic toxicity.
B. Post–traumatic brain injury (TBI).
C. Hepatic encephalopathy.
D. Alcohol withdrawal.
E. Hypoxia.

The correct response is option D.

A low-voltage fast activity EEG finding is consistent with alcohol withdrawal or benzodiazepine intoxication.

Diffuse slowing on the EEG, the most common presentation in delirium, is suggestive of an etiology involving anticholinergic toxicity, posttraumatic brain injury, hepatic encephalopathy, or hypoxia. **(p. 476 [Table 11–8])**

11.10 Delirium rating scales are useful in the diagnosis and monitoring of delirium symptoms. Which of the following statements about the Memorial Delirium Assessment Scale (MDAS) is *false?*

A. It is a severity rating scale designed to be used after a delirium diagnosis has been made.
B. It allows for repeated ratings.
C. Items on the MDAS specifically address temporal onset and symptom fluctuation.
D. The MDAS correlates highly with the Delirium Rating Scale.
E. It has been found useful in distinguishing delirium from other psychiatric illnesses in elderly patients.

The correct response is option C.

The MDAS does not include items addressing temporal onset and fluctuation of symptoms, which are characteristic symptoms that help to distinguish delirium from dementia.

The MDAS is a 10-item severity rating scale for use after a diagnosis of delirium has been made. It was intended for repeated ratings within a 24-hour period. The MDAS correlates highly with the Delirium Rating Scale and the Mini-Mental State Examination. The Japanese version of the MDAS was validated in 37 elderly patients with delirium, dementia, mood disorder, or schizophrenia and was found to reliably distinguish among the disorders (Matsuoka et al. 2001). **(p. 473)**

References

American Psychiatric Association: Diagnostic and Statistical Manual: Mental Disorders. Washington, DC, American Psychiatric Association, 1952

American Psychiatric Association: Diagnostic and Statistical Manual of Mental Disorders, 2nd Edition. Washington, DC, American Psychiatric Association, 1968

American Psychiatric Association: Diagnostic and Statistical Manual of Mental Disorders, 3rd Edition. Washington, DC, American Psychiatric Association, 1980

American Psychiatric Association: Diagnostic and Statistical Manual of Mental Disorders, 3rd Edition, Revised. Washington, DC, American Psychiatric Association, 1987

American Psychiatric Association: Diagnostic and Statistical Manual of Mental Disorders, 4th Edition. Washington, DC, American Psychiatric Association, 1994

Matsuoka Y, Miyake Y, Arakaki H, et al: Clinical utility and validation of the Japanese version of the Memorial Delirium Assessment Scale in a psychogeriatric inpatient setting. Gen Hosp Psychiatry 23:36–40, 2001

Trzepacz PT, Mittal D, Torres R, et al: Delirium vs dementia symptoms: Delirium Rating Scale—Revised (DRS-R-98) and Cognitive Test for Delirium (CTD) item comparisons. Psychosomatics 43:156–157, 2002

CHAPTER 12

Neuropsychiatric Aspects of Aphasia and Related Disorders

Select the single best response for each question.

12.1 The current classification of aphasia syndromes is based on the Wernicke-Geschwind model, which posits that aphasia involves six major language areas. Which of the following is *not* one of the language areas addressed in this model?

A. Fluency.
B. Spelling.
C. Naming.
D. Repetition.
E. Reading.

The correct response is option B.

Spelling is not a major language area according to the Wernicke-Geschwind model.

Classification of aphasia syndromes by this model requires the examination of six major language areas: fluency, confrontational naming, auditory comprehension, repetition, reading, and writing. **(p. 521)**

12.2 In which of the following aphasia syndromes is auditory comprehension abnormal?

A. Anomia.
B. Broca's.
C. Conduction.
D. Transcortical motor.
E. Wernicke's.

The correct response is option E.

Auditory comprehension is abnormal in Wernicke's aphasia, as well as in global aphasia and transcortical sensory aphasia.

Auditory comprehension is relatively normal in anomia, Broca's aphasia, conduction aphasia, and transcortical motor aphasia. **(p. 522 [Table 12–1])**

12.3 In Broca's aphasia, which of the following language areas is relatively normal?

A. Auditory comprehension.
B. Fluency.
C. Naming.
D. Repetition.
E. Writing comprehension.

The correct response is option A.

In Broca's aphasia, auditory comprehension is relatively normal.

Fluency, naming, repetition, and writing comprehension are all abnormal in Broca's aphasia, and reading can be either normal or abnormal. **(p. 522 [Table 12–1])**

12.4 Patients with delirium typically exhibit abnormalities in all of the following language functions *except*

A. Writing.
B. Word-list generation.
C. Motor speech.
D. Automatic speech.
E. Content of speech.

The correct response is option D.

Automatic speech is normal in patients suffering from delirium.

Patients with delirium commonly exhibit abnormal writing and word-list generation, dysarthric and incoherent motor speech, and incoherent speech content. **(p. 525 [Table 12–2])**

12.5 Which of the following language areas is relatively normal in transcortical motor aphasia but abnormal in Broca's aphasia?

A. Fluency.
B. Naming.
C. Repetition.
D. Writing comprehension.
E. Reading.

The correct response is option C.

Transcortical motor aphasia resembles Broca's aphasia in its decreased verbal fluency but differs in the relatively preserved ability to repeat spoken language. Thus, patients with transcortical motor aphasia may struggle to utter words in spontaneous conversation that they can easily say on repetition. **(p. 525)**

12.6 Nonfluent (anterior) aphasia and fluent (posterior) aphasia each are accompanied by a distinct, long-term behavioral syndrome. In anterior aphasia behavioral syndrome, the most common psychiatric symptom is

A. Agitation.
B. Depression.
C. Paranoia.
D. Suicide.
E. Impulsive behavior.

The correct response is option B.

Depression is considerably more common and intense in patients with anterior aphasia, due in part to these patients' ability to recognize their impairment and their frustration with not being able to express their thoughts and desires.

Paranoia, agitation, impulsivity, and suicidal behavior are all much more common in patients with posterior aphasia. These patients have difficulty comprehending spoken language and remain unaware of their deficit, producing a persistent unconcern that is pathological. **(pp. 529–530)**

CHAPTER 13

Neuropsychiatric Aspects of Aggression and Impulse-Control Disorders

Select the single best response for each question.

13.1 Which of the following statements regarding violence in the United States is *false*?

A. Homicide is the second leading cause of death among persons 15–24 years of age.
B. Half of all homicides are committed by perpetrators younger than 25 years.
C. The rate of homicide death for men is three times that for women.
D. In domestic violence, men are more likely than women to attack a spouse.
E. In 90% of homicides, perpetrator and victim are of the same race.

The correct response is option D.

In domestic violence, wives are more likely to attack their husbands than vice versa.

In the United States, homicide is the second leading cause of death among individuals 15–24 years of age; homicide remains the leading cause of death among black men and women 15–34 years of age. In 90% of homicides, the perpetrator and victim are the same race. A greater percentage of the aggression in our society is associated with the young: half of all homicides are committed by those younger than age 25 years. Overall, rates of death by homicide are about three times greater for men than for women. **(p. 536)**

13.2 Which of the following is the interview instrument most commonly used to evaluate aggression?

A. Buss-Durkee Hostility Inventory.
B. Hostility and Direction of Hostility Questionnaire.
C. Spielberger State-Trait Anger Expression Inventory.
D. Barratt Impulsiveness Scale.
E. Brown-Goodwin Assessment.

The correct response is option A.

The most widely used self-report assessment of aggression is the Buss-Durkee Hostility Inventory, a 75-item true/false questionnaire that measures different aspects of hostility, aggression, and danger. There are eight subscales: assault, indirect hostility, irritability, negativism, resentment, suspicion, verbal hostility, and guilt.

Other commonly used self-report instruments include the Hostility and Direction of Hostility Questionnaire, a 51-item true/false questionnaire that contains five subscales, of which only one, "acting out hostility," is relevant to aggressive behavior; the Spielberger State-Trait Anger Expression Inventory, a 44-item scale that divides behavior into state anger and trait anger; and the Barratt

Impulsiveness Scale, a 30-item scale that assesses long-term patterns of behavior by asking subjects questions about the way they think and act without relation to any specified time period. The Brown-Goodwin Assessment for Life History of Aggression, one of the most widely used interview instruments, is rated by a clinician based on direct interview with the patient and/or a review of medical records. It contains 11 assessments of aggression: temper, fighting, assault, school discipline, civilian discipline, antisocial behavior not involving police, antisocial behavior involving police, military discipline, military judicial discipline, property damage, and verbal aggression. **(pp. 537–538)**

13.3 The hypothalamus has been the focus of much research on the neurobiology of aggression. Which of the following statements is *true*?

A. Stimulation of the anterior hypothalamus in cats produces submissive behavior.
B. Stimulation of the dorsomedial hypothalamus in the cat causes increased predatory attacks on small animals.
C. Lesioning of the ventromedial nucleus in cats results in permanent aggression.
D. Stimulation of the posterior lateral aspect of the hypothalamus in cats prolongs latency of attack.
E. Stimulation of the medial ventral area of the hypothalamus shortens latency of attack.

The correct response is option C.

Destruction of aggression-inhibitory areas, such as the ventromedial nucleus of the hypothalamus, produces permanently aggressive cats and rats.

The hypothalamus plays a major role in the expression of aggression in animals. Stimulation of the anterior hypothalamus in cats produces predatory attacks. Stimulation of the dorsomedial aspects produces aggression in which the animal ignores the presence of a rat and attacks the experimenter. Stimulation of the posterior lateral aspect produces a posture of preparation for attack. Stimulation of the medial ventral area prolongs the latency of the attack. **(p. 540)**

13.4 In primates, bilateral temporal lobectomy produces the Klüver-Bucy syndrome, which is characterized by all of the following behaviors *except*

A. Hyperorality.
B. Hyposexuality.
C. Absence of fear response.
D. Increased touching.
E. Visual agnosia.

The correct response is option B.

Bilateral temporal lobectomy does not produce hyposexuality, but rather *hyper*sexuality, along with hyperorality, absence of fear response, increased touching , and visual agnosia. **(p. 541)**

13.5 Which of the following statements regarding serotonin and impulsive aggression is *true*?

A. There is a positive relationship between violent lethal suicidal behavior and 5-hydroxyindoleacetic acid (5-HIAA) in depressed patients.
B. Homicide offenders with a suicide attempt history have a higher concentration of cerebrospinal fluid (CSF) 5-HIAA compared with those without a history of suicide attempts.
C. Low CSF 5-HIAA is related to aggressive behavior independent of suicidal behavior in patient with Axis I disorders.
D. Increased brain stem levels of serotonin and 5-HIAA are found in suicide victims.
E. Increased platelet serotonin receptor sites are found in aggressive subjects.

The correct response is option C.

Low CSF 5-HIAA is related to aggressive behavior independent of suicidal behavior in patients with Axis I disorders.

There is a negative relationship between violent suicidal behavior and 5-HIAA in depressed patients. Homicide offenders with a history of suicide attempts have lower concentrations of 5-HIAA than do those without such a history. Decreased brain stem levels of serotonin and 5-HIAA have been found in postmortem studies of suicide victims. Decreased platelet serotonin transporter sites are found in aggressive subjects with conduct disorder. **(pp. 542, 544)**

13.6 A number of inborn metabolic disorders are associated with aggressive and impulsive behavior. Which of the following inherited illnesses is characterized by increased mucopolysaccharide storage?

A. Sanfilippo's syndrome.
B. Phenylketonuria.
C. Lesch-Nyhan syndrome.
D. Prader-Willi syndrome.
E. Vogt's syndrome.

The correct response is option A.

Sanfilippo's syndrome is associated with increased mucopolysaccharide storage.

Phenylketonuria is a genetic disorder in which the body is unable to utilize an essential amino acid, phenylalanine. Lesch-Nyhan syndrome is a rare, inherited disorder caused by a deficiency of the enzyme hypoxanthine-guanine phosphoribosyltransferase. Prader-Willi syndrome is a genetic disorder in which seven genes (or some subset thereof) on chromosome 15 are missing or unexpressed (chromosome 15q partial deletion) on the paternal chromosome. Vogt's syndrome is a neuronal storage disorder. **(p. 547)**

13.7 Neuropsychological testing has revealed correlations between laterality of cerebral dysfunction and specific clinical profiles. On testing, which of the following clinical subgroups shows predominantly right hemisphere dysfunction?

A. Alcoholic individuals with affective disorders.
B. Violent criminals.
C. Alcoholic individuals with personality disorders.
D. Adolescents with conduct disorders.
E. Prisoners with impulsive behaviors.

The correct response is option A.

Using the Halstead-Reitan battery, Yeudall and Fromm-Auch (1979) studied laterality of cerebral dysfunction in various subject groups. They found impairments on variables sensitive primarily to left hemisphere dysfunction in violent criminals, alcoholic individuals with personality disorders, and adolescents with conduct disorders, but predominantly right hemisphere dysfunction in nonviolent criminals, alcoholic individuals with affective disorders, and individuals with affective personality disorders. Fedora and Fedora (1983) also found that prisoners with impulsive behaviors had evidence of left hemisphere impairment. **(p. 551)**

13.8 Which of the following personality disorders has been found to be common in arsonists?

A. Narcissistic.
B. Histrionic.
C. Schizoid.
D. Borderline.
E. Avoidant.

The correct response is option D.

In a study by Virkkunen et al. (1987), all of the arsonists met DSM-III (American Psychiatric Association 1980) criteria for borderline personality disorder. **(p. 552)**

13.9 Which of the following selective serotonin reuptake inhibitors (SSRIs) has been most extensively studied for the treatment of impulsivity and aggression in borderline personality disorder?

A. Fluvoxamine.
B. Fluoxetine.
C. Sertraline.
D. Citalopram.
E. Paroxetine.

The correct response is option B.

Fluoxetine is the best-studied SSRI for the treatment of impulsivity and aggression. **(pp. 552–553)**

References

American Psychiatric Association: Diagnostic and Statistical Manual of Mental Disorders, 3rd Edition. Washington, DC, American Psychiatric Association, 1980

Fedora O, Fedora S: Some neuropsychological and psychophysiological aspects of psychopathic and nonpsychopathic criminals, in Laterality and Psychopathology. Edited by Flor-Henry P, Gruzelier J. Amsterdam, Elsevier, 1983, pp 20–25

Virkkunen M, Nuutila A, Goodwin FK, et al: Cerebrospinal fluid monoamine metabolite levels in male arsonists. Arch Gen Psychiatry 44:241–247, 1987

Yeudall LT, Fromm-Auch D: Neuropsychological impairments in various psychopathological populations, in Hemisphere Asymmetries of Function in Psychopathology. Edited by Gruzelier J, Flor-Henry P. Amsterdam, Elsevier, 1979, pp 81–83

CHAPTER 14

Neuropsychiatric Aspects of Memory and Amnesia

Select the single best response for each question.

14.1 All of the following statements concerning declarative memory are true *except*

A. It is the type of memory assessed by traditional tests of recall and recognition.
B. It is defined as the conscious recollection of words, scenes, faces, stories, and events.
C. It encompasses the subordinate functions of procedural memory, classical conditioning, simple associative learning, and priming.
D. It is usually subdivided into two components: semantic and episodic memory.
E. Its functioning depends on the integrity of the hippocampus and related structures.

The correct response is option C.

Procedural memory, classical conditioning, simple associative learning, and priming are *not* subsumed under the heading of declarative memory; rather, these types of memory belong under the heading of *non*declarative memory.

Declarative memory describes the conscious recollection of words, scenes, faces, stories, and events. It is the type of memory assessed by traditional tests of recall and recognition, which rely on what has been called the explicit retrieval of information. Declarative memory is usually subdivided into two components: semantic and episodic memory. *Semantic memory* refers to the acquisition of factual information about the world. *Episodic memory* refers to the recording and conscious recollection of personal experiences. Declarative memory is dependent on the integrity of the hippocampus and its related structures. **(pp. 567, 568)**

14.2 Working memory…

A. Is a form of nondeclarative memory.
B. Is viewed as a single memory buffer.
C. Is a form of declarative memory.
D. Has the central executive as its most important component.
E. Is similar to what in the past was called *long-term memory*.

The correct response is option D.

The central executive is presumably the most important component of working memory, although its role is the least well defined. One of its functions is to coordinate information from the separate subsystems.

Working memory is typically perceived as distinct from the declarative and nondeclarative memory systems. It is viewed not as a single memory buffer, but instead as three interrelated components: an attention controller (the *central executive*) aided by two active "slave" subsystems, the articulatory or phonological loop and the visuospatial "scratch pad" or "sketch pad." **(pp. 567–568, 570)**

14.3 Clinical characteristics commonly observed in amnesic patients include all of the following *except*

A. Anterograde amnesia.
B. Aphasia.
C. Retrograde amnesia.
D. Confabulations.
E. Intact intellectual function.

The correct response is option B.

Aphasia is not a clinical characteristic typically found in amnesic patients.

Four clinical characteristics are typical of most amnesic patients: anterograde amnesia, retrograde amnesia, confabulation, and intact intellectual function. *Anterograde amnesia* is the hallmark of an amnesic disorder and refers to the inability to acquire new information for explicit retrieval. *Retrograde amnesia* refers to difficulty in retrieving events that occurred before the onset of the amnesic disorder. *Confabulation* is providing made-up or inaccurate information without having any apparent awareness that the response is incorrect. Intellectual function remains relatively intact in classic amnesic disorders, although some specific secondary cognitive defects may be noted on careful neuropsychological testing. **(p. 572)**

14.4 Depressed patients are more likely than nondepressed patients to have deficits in which of the following domains?

A. Effortful processing.
B. Automatic processing.
C. Nondeclarative memory.
D. Incidental learning.
E. None of the above.

The correct response is option A.

In general, depressed patients are more likely to manifest deficits on tasks that require effort or greater depth of processing, but not on tasks that can be completed automatically. Committing to memory a long shopping list is an example of effortful processing that may be impaired in depressed patients.

Depressed patients tend to have deficits in the declarative but not the nondeclarative domain. This pattern may be useful clinically to distinguish depressed patients from those with Alzheimer's disease. Our learning and retaining what we had for breakfast—that is, incidental learning—is an example of automatic processing that is usually normal in depressed patients. **(pp. 576–577)**

14.5 All of the following statements concerning declarative memory deficits in patients with schizophrenia are true *except*

A. Deficits are more pronounced in tests of recognition than in tests of recall.
B. Patients usually have little or no deficits in nondeclarative memory tests.
C. Procedural learning is usually intact with few or no deficits.
D. Patients have shallow or inefficient encoding of information.
E. Patients frequently exhibit disorganized or inefficient retrieval strategies.

The correct response is option A.

Declarative memory deficits in schizophrenia are usually more pronounced in tests of recall than in tests of recognition.

In schizophrenic patients, there is little or no deficit in nondeclarative memory tasks, including procedural memory (as reflected in motor skill learning) and implicit memory (as reflected in various tests of perceptual and conceptual priming). The deficits in explicit recall have often been attributed to shallow or inefficient encoding of information, disorganized or inefficient retrieval strategies, and rapid forgetting. **(p. 579)**

14.6 Which of the following statements concerning dissociative amnesia is *true*?

A. It is frequently diagnosed, especially among patients with "hysterical" disorders.
B. It usually interferes with social or occupational functioning.
C. It is more common in males.
D. It is more common in the elderly than in adolescents or young adults.
E. It usually is transient.

The correct response is option E.

Dissociative amnesia is usually transient; most cases show rapid recovery of memory.

Dissociative amnesia is rarely diagnosed, even among patients who receive a diagnosis of "hysterical" disorders, since it does not necessarily interfere with social or occupational functioning. Furthermore, patients with dissociative amnesia may display indifference to their symptomatology and thus be unlikely to seek treatment. Dissociative amnesia is more common among females, and it is thought to occur more often in adolescents and young adults than in the elderly. **(p. 580)**

14.7 All of the following medications may adversely affect memory *except*

A. Benzodiazepines.
B. Heterocyclic antidepressants.
C. Neuroleptics.
D. Atypical antipsychotics.
E. Antiparkinsonian agents.

The correct response is option D.

Although the evidence is still circumstantial and tentative, it appears that atypical antipsychotic agents have an ameliorative effect on cognitive deficits in schizophrenia, with risperidone exerting stronger beneficial effects on working (short-term) memory and olanzapine exerting stronger action on verbal learning and memory.

Benzodiazepines have a deleterious effect on memory, with the most characteristic deficit being diminished delayed recall for newly learned information. A wide range of medications have anticholinergic properties, including heterocyclic antidepressants, neuroleptics, and antiparkinsonian agents. Anticholinergics can produce sedation, attentional impairment, memory disturbance, and, in extreme cases, an anticholinergic delirium. **(pp. 583–584)**

CHAPTER 15

Neuropsychiatric Aspects of Traumatic Brain Injury

Select the single best response for each question.

15.1 Traumatic brain injury (TBI) is associated with profound perturbations of neurotransmitters. Which of the following statements regarding post-TBI neurotransmitter changes is *false*?

A. Excitotoxicity following TBI is mediated by glutamate and acetylcholine.
B. Acute elevations of striatal dopamine post-TBI predict poor functional recovery.
C. Decreased levels of 5-hydroxyindoleacetic acid (5-HIAA) are found with frontotemporal contusions.
D. Decreased levels of 5-HIAA are found with diffuse contusions.
E. TBI is associated acutely with an increase in cholinergic transmission.

The correct response is option D.

Increased levels of 5-HIAA are found in patients with diffuse contusions, while decreased levels of 5-HIAA are present in patients with frontotemporal contusions.

Acute elevations of striatal dopamine are predictive of poor recovery from TBI. Traumatic brain injury appears to produce an acute increase in cholinergic neurotransmission followed by chronic reduction in neurotransmitter function and cholinergic afferents. **(pp. 597, 598)**

15.2 A traumatic brain injury (TBI) patient with eye opening to speech (but not spontaneously), decorticate motor response, and intelligible but incoherent speech would score ___ on the Glasgow Coma Scale.

A. 8.
B. 9.
C. 10.
D. 11.
E. 12.

The correct response is option B.

That patient would score 9 on the Glasgow Coma Scale. **(p. 600; Table 15–3)**

15.3 Traumatic brain injury (TBI) affecting the frontal lobe is common. Damage to specific frontal lobe regions is associated with particular behavior symptoms. All of the following symptoms are characteristic of the orbitofrontal syndrome *except*

A. Perseveration.
B. Impulsivity.
C. Disinhibition.
D. Hyperactivity.
E. Mood lability.

The correct response is option A.

Perseveration is not a characteristic of orbitofrontal syndrome, but is seen with injury to the dorsolateral frontal cortex. The orbitofrontal syndrome is associated with behavioral excesses, such as impulsivity, disinhibition, hyperactivity, distractibility, and mood lability. **(p. 607)**

15.4 Post–traumatic brain injury (TBI) epilepsy presents a clinical challenge, in that several anticonvulsants are themselves associated with impaired cognitive function. Among the following anticonvulsants used to treat post-TBI epilepsy, which is *least* likely to cause adverse effects on cognition?

A. Phenytoin.
B. Carbamazepine.
C. Topiramate.
D. Lamotrigine.
E. Phenobarbital.

The correct response is option D.

Among the newer anticonvulsant medications, lamotrigine has demonstrated fewer adverse cognitive effects than topiramate.

Among the older anticonvulsant agents, phenytoin, carbamazepine, and phenobarbital have all demonstrated adverse effects on cognitive performance. Phenytoin has more profound effects on cognition than does carbamazepine; however, both phenytoin and carbamazepine have negative effects on cognitive function, especially on tasks that involve motor and speed performance. Intellectual deterioration in children undergoing long-term treatment with phenytoin or phenobarbital has also been documented. **(p. 613)**

15.5 Post–traumatic brain injury (TBI) aggression often exhibits distinctive behavioral features. Which of the following content/context descriptors does *not* characterize the violence committed by these patients?

A. Reactive.
B. Nonreflective.
C. Nonpurposeful.
D. Periodic.
E. Ego-syntonic.

The correct response is option E.

In patients who exhibit aggressive behavior after brain injury, the aggression is ego-*dystonic,* such that the individual is often upset or embarrassed after the episode.

Typically, the violence seen in post-TBI patients is reactive (i.e., triggered by modest or trivial stimuli); nonreflective, in that it does not involve premeditation or planning; nonpurposeful, in the sense that the aggression serves no obvious long-term goal; and periodic, with brief outbursts of rage and aggression interspersed between long periods of relatively calm behavior. **(pp. 616, 617)**

15.6 Clinical guidelines for psychopharmacological treatment of the psychiatric sequelae of traumatic brain injury (TBI) include all of the following *except*

A. Start low (dose) and go slow (with dosage escalations).
B. Continuously reassess clinical status.
C. Monitor for drug–drug interactions.
D. Augment partial responses.
E. Limit doses to less than usual full recommended doses.

The correct response is option E.

Because patients with brain injury of any type are far more sensitive to the side effects of medications than are patients who do not have brain injury, doses of psychotropic medications must be raised or lowered in small increments over protracted periods of time. However, patients ultimately may require the same doses and serum levels that are therapeutically effective for patients without brain injury.

Several general guidelines should be followed in the pharmacological treatment of the psychiatric syndromes that occur after TBI: 1) start low, go slow, 2) conduct a therapeutic trial of all medications, 3) maintain continuous reassessment of the clinical condition, 4) monitor drug–drug interactions, 5) augment partial response, and 6) discontinue or lower the dose of the most recently prescribed medication if there is a worsening of the treated symptom soon after the medication had been initiated (or increased). **(p. 618)**

15.7 Pathological laughing and/or crying (PLC) is a classic disorder of affective dysregulation that is an infrequent consequence of traumatic brain injury (TBI). Which of the following statements about PLC is *false*?

A. Episodes of crying and/or laughter do not produce a persistent change in mood.
B. Episodes may occur many times a day.
C. Episodes must be provoked by emotionally evocative stimuli.
D. Presentation of symptoms is quite stereotyped.
E. Episodes are uncontrollable.

The correct response is option C.

In PLC, the episodes of involuntary crying and/or laughing are often provoked by trivial (i.e., not sentimental) stimuli, may occur many times per day, are quite stereotyped in their presentation, are uncontrollable, do not evoke a concordant subjective affective experience, and do not produce a persistent change in the prevailing mood. **(p. 621)**

15.8 Atypical antipsychotics are commonly used in management of the behavioral consequences of traumatic brain injury (TBI). However, the physician must be mindful of adverse drug effects in this vulnerable population. Among the following atypical antipsychotics, which is the *least* likely to produce extrapyramidal side effects (EPS)?

A. Risperidone.
B. Ziprasidone.
C. Quetiapine.
D. Olanzapine.
E. Aripiprazole.

The correct response is option C.

Among the newer atypical antipsychotic medications, quetiapine produces the fewest EPS.

Risperidone, olanzapine, aripiprazole, and ziprasidone may all have a role in the treatment of post-TBI psychosis, but published literature on them is limited. **(pp. 623–624)**

15.9 Which of the following classes of medications is *not* recommended for use in chronically agitated traumatic brain injury (TBI) patients?

A. β-Blockers.
B. Buspirone.
C. Serotonergic antidepressants.
D. Atypical antipsychotics.
E. Benzodiazepines.

The correct response is option E.

Benzodiazepines are not recommended for treatment of chronic agitation; however, they may be needed acutely for temporary sedation in cases of severe agitation or aggression in post-TBI patients.

β-Blockers, buspirone, serotonergic antidepressants (e.g., selective serotonin reuptake inhibitors, trazodone), atypical antipsychotics, and anticonvulsants are indicated for chronic agitation. **(pp. 627, 628; Table 15–13)**

CHAPTER 16

Neuropsychiatric Aspects of Seizure Disorders

Select the single best response for each question.

16.1 The International League Against Epilepsy (ILAE) has proposed a five-axis diagnostic scheme to classify seizures. Which of the five axes is used to specify etiology?

A. Axis I.
B. Axis II.
C. Axis III.
D. Axis IV.
E. Axis V.

The correct response is option D.

In the ILAE proposed diagnostic scheme (International League Against Epilepsy Commission Report 2001a, 2001b), Axis IV is used to classify etiology (when etiology is known). The physician specifies genetic defects or specific pathologies from the ILAE Classification of Diseases Frequently Associated With Epileptic Seizures or Epilepsy Syndromes.

Axis I is used to record ictal phenomenology (a description of the ictal events). Axis II is used to record seizure type. The physician specifies the type from the ILAE List of Epileptic Seizures, identifying localization within the brain or precipitating stimuli when appropriate. Axis III is used to record the type of epileptic syndrome (when a syndrome diagnosis is possible). The physician specifies the syndrome type from the ILAE List of Epilepsy Syndromes. Axis V is used to record World Health Organization impairment classifications. **(pp. 650–651; Table 16–2)**

16.2 In which of the following seizure types is consciousness preserved?

A. Tonic-clonic seizures.
B. Simple partial seizures.
C. Status epilepticus.
D. Absence seizures.
E. Complex partial seizures.

The correct response is option B.

In *simple partial seizures* (previously called *elementary partial seizures*), no alteration in consciousness is present. Simple partial seizures are a form of *focal seizures* (also called partial or localization-related seizures), which are so named because epileptic firing starts in a specific focus in the brain, usually the cerebral cortex.

Tonic-clonic seizures (or grand mal seizures) are the most common form of generalized seizure. They manifest as total loss of consciousness with a tetanic muscular phase, followed by a phase of repetitive jerking. *Status epilepticus* is a continuous seizure state that involves two or more seizures superimposed on each other without total recovery of consciousness and is a true medical emergency. *Generalized status epilepticus* can be convulsive, consisting of tonic-clonic seizures, or nonconvulsive. *Absence seizures* (or petit mal seizures) occur primarily in children, are generalized from the start, and involve loss of consciousness for a few seconds without any motor phase. *Complex partial seizures* are another form of focal seizures. They involve a defect in consciousness, usually confusion and dizziness. **(pp. 651–652)**

16.3 Which of the following is the major laboratory test used in the diagnostic workup of seizures?

A. Prolactin level.
B. Serum albumin.
C. Serum potassium.
D. Serum calcium.
E. Creatine phosphokinase (CPK).

The correct response is option A.

Prolactin level is the only major laboratory test used in the diagnostic workup of seizures. A hormone secreted by the anterior pituitary gland, serum prolactin, is released by epileptic activity spreading from the temporal lobe to the hypothalamic-pituitary axis. After a seizure, usually within 15–20 minutes after a generalized tonic-clonic seizure, there will be an abrupt rise in prolactin levels. As a rule, the prolactin level decreases to normal within 60 minutes; therefore, blood should be drawn 15–20 minutes after the seizure. These levels are typically three to four times the patient's baseline prolactin level. This response of prolactin is seen more often in major motor seizures and less frequently in partial complex seizures. **(p. 654)**

16.4 Which of the following statements about nonepileptic seizures (pseudoseizures) is *false*?

A. Injury is infrequent.
B. Plantar flexor reflexes are preserved.
C. Postictal features are typical.
D. Sleep-related seizures are infrequent.
E. Restraint accentuates the seizure.

The correct response is option C.

Postictal features are not present in nonepileptic seizures, also known as *pseudoseizures*.

The term *nonepileptic seizure* is used synonymously with *pseudoseizure* or *conversion reaction*. Patients with nonepileptic seizures differ from seizure disorder patients in that they may have significantly more stress, more negative life events, and a history of child abuse, and they often have more somatic symptoms and more awareness of their bodies. Most patients with nonepileptic seizures demonstrate somatoform disorders, particularly conversion, rather than dissociative disorders. A significant number of patients with nonepileptic seizures also suffer from concomitant mood and anxiety disorders. For this reason, combination treatment with psychotropic medications such as selective serotonin reuptake inhibitors, benzodiazepines, and atypical antipsychotics and individual psychotherapy can be extremely helpful in reducing the frequency of and morbidity associated with nonepileptic seizures. **(pp. 656, 657 [Table 16–7])**

16.5 Which of the following diagnostic clues may help differentiate psychosis due to a central nervous system lesion or seizures from schizophrenic psychosis?

A. Presentation that meets DSM-IV (American Psychiatric Association 1994) criteria.
B. Poor premorbid social history.
C. Gradual change in personality, mood, or ability to function.
D. Rapid fluctuations in mental status.
E. Responsiveness to usual biological or psychological interventions.

The correct response is option D.

Rapid fluctuations in mental status are indicative of a lesion of the central nervous system or of seizures.

Other clues are a presentation that does not meet DSM-IV criteria for schizophrenia, a good premorbid social history, and an abrupt change in personality, mood, or ability to function. Patients with a seizure disorder and psychosis often talk about their symptoms in almost a detached manner. Most of the patients seem quite intact even when experiencing the symptoms, particularly between episodes. In addition, the usual pharmacological or psychotherapeutic treatments for psychosis are not effective. **(pp. 660–661; Table 16–8)**

16.6 Basic guidelines for treating seizure disorder patients with concomitant psychiatric symptoms include all of the following *except*

A. Preferably use anticonvulsant monotherapy.
B. Start with higher doses of psychotropic medications in order to rapidly treat symptoms.
C. Anticipate possible drug interactions between anticonvulsant and psychotropic medications.
D. Evaluate the need for adjustment of the anticonvulsant.
E. Optimize the addition of psychotropic medication by targeting specific psychiatric symptoms.

The correct response is option B.

The psychiatrist should start with lower, not higher, doses of psychotropic medication and should wait until symptoms stabilize before changing doses.

After performing a thorough assessment of the biopsychosocial factors that can aggravate the neuropsychiatric symptoms of the seizure disorder patient and evaluating the need for adjustment of the anticonvulsant, the psychiatrist should preferably use anticonvulsant monotherapy. Psychotherapeutic approaches (individual, family, group) that are specific for the syndrome or that target behaviors or stressors should be considered, and interactions between anticonvulsant and psychotropic medications should be anticipated. **(p. 667 [Table 16–10])**

References

American Psychiatric Association: Diagnostic and Statistical Manual of Mental Disorders, 4th Edition. Washington, DC, American Psychiatric Association, 1994

International League Against Epilepsy Commission Report: Glossary of descriptive terminology for ictal semiology: report of the ILAE task force on classification and terminology. Epilepsia 42:1212–1218, 2001a

International League Against Epilepsy Commission Report: A proposed diagnostic scheme for people with epileptic seizures and with epilepsy: report of the ILAE Task Force on Classification and Terminology. Epilepsia 42:796–803, 2001b

CHAPTER 17

Neuropsychiatric Aspects of Sleep and Sleep Disorders

Select the single best response for each question.

17.1 Sleep stages are defined by specific electroencephalographic parameters. Which sleep stage features sleep spindles or K complexes, with high-amplitude delta activity for less than 20% of the epoch?

A. Stage I.
B. Stage II.
C. Stage III.
D. Stage IV.
E. Rapid eye movement (REM).

The correct response is option B.

Stage II is scored when sleep spindles or K complexes occur and high-amplitude delta electroencephalographic activity occupies less than 20% of an epoch.

If there is 20%–50% delta activity, Stage III is designated, and if there is more than 50% delta activity, the epoch is classified as sleep Stage IV. Stage I is an intermediate non-alpha state characterized by low-voltage, mixed-frequency electroencephalographic activity that is deltaless; it is a spindleless stage that does not have K complexes. Stages I, II, III, and IV are sometimes collectively referred to as non-REM (NREM) sleep. Stages III and IV are often combined and called slow-wave sleep (SWS). **(p. 678)**

17.2 Which of the following general statements about sleep architecture is *false*?

A. Sleep is entered through non–rapid eye movement (NREM) sleep.
B. NREM and rapid eye movement (REM) sleep alternate every 90 minutes.
C. Slow-wave sleep dominates the first third of the night.
D. REM sleep dominates the last third of the night.
E. REM episodes are shorter later in the sleep period.

The correct response is option E.

REM sleep occurs in 4–6 discrete episodes each night, with episodes generally being longer later in the sleep period.

Sleep is entered through NREM sleep, and NREM and REM sleep alternate approximately every 90 minutes. Slow-wave sleep predominates during the first third of the night, and REM sleep predominates during the last third of the night. **(p. 680)**

17.3 Sleep disturbances in major depression include all of the following *except*

A. Generalized sleep disturbance.
B. Increase in slow-wave sleep in the first non–rapid eye movement (NREM)–rapid eye movement (REM) cycle.
C. Lengthening of latency to REM sleep.
D. Occurrence of REM sleep earlier in the night.
E. Increase in REM density.

The correct response is option C.

REM latency is shortened, not lengthened, in sleep disturbances in depressed patients.

Sleep disturbances in major depression include generalized sleep disturbance (increased sleep latency, increased nocturnal awakening, and early-morning awakenings), decrease in slow-wave sleep during the first NREM–REM cycle, shortening of latency to REM sleep, occurrence of REM sleep earlier in the night, and increase in REM density, especially early in the night. Interestingly, most antidepressant medications—including selective serotonin reuptake inhibitors, tricyclic antidepressants, and monoamine oxidase inhibitors—suppress REM sleep. **(p. 683)**

17.4 Although most antidepressants are known to suppress rapid eye movement (REM) sleep, some antidepressants do not have this property. Which of the following antidepressants does not suppress REM sleep?

A. Paroxetine.
B. Fluoxetine.
C. Desipramine.
D. Monoamine oxidase inhibitors.
E. Bupropion.

The correct response is option E.

Bupropion does not suppress REM sleep, and neither does nefazodone. Most antidepressants (including selective serotonin reuptake inhibitors, tricyclic antidepressants, and monoamine oxidase inhibitors) suppress REM sleep. **(p. 683)**

17.5 Psychophysiological insomnia is a troubling sleep disorder with specific behavioral characteristics. Which of the following is *not* a feature of this condition?

A. Excessive worry about not being able to sleep.
B. Trying too hard to sleep.
C. Rumination.
D. Inability to sleep unless in one's own bed.
E. Increased muscle tension when retiring.

The correct response is option D.

Psychophysiological insomnia does *not* feature inability to sleep unless in one's own bed; in fact, patients with this condition sleep better away from their own bedrooms, including in the sleep laboratory. Features of psychophysiological insomnia include excessive worry about not being able to sleep, trying too hard to sleep, rumination, inability to clear one's mind while trying to sleep, increased muscle tension when getting into bed, other somatic manifestations of anxiety, and ability to fall asleep when not trying (e.g., when watching TV). **(p. 686)**

17.6 Disorders of daytime sleepiness can cause great functional impairment and even physically dangerous behavior. Which of the following is the most common cause of excessive daytime sleepiness?

A. Sleep apnea.
B. Narcolepsy.
C. Idiopathic hypersomnia.
D. Kleine-Levin syndrome.
E. Posttraumatic hypersomnia.

The correct response is option A.

Sleep apnea accounts for 43.2% of disorders associated with excessive daytime sleepiness.

The two next most common sleep disorders producing hypersomnia are narcolepsy and idiopathic hypersomnia, followed by recurrent hypersomnia, or Kleine-Levin syndrome, and posttraumatic hypersomnia resulting from brain or brain stem injury. **(p. 694)**

17.7 Predisposing factors for obstructive sleep apnea include all of the following *except*

A. Hyperthyroidism and acromegaly.
B. Male sex.
C. Middle age or older.
D. Obesity.
E. Micrognathia or retrognathia.

The correct response is option A.

Hypothyroidism and acromegaly are predisposing factors for obstructive sleep apnea.

Clinical features associated with obstructive sleep apnea include excessive daytime sleepiness; loud snoring with frequent awakening; awakening with choking and/or gasping for breath, morning dry mouth; and witnessed apnea. Predisposing factors include male sex, middle age, obesity, micrognathia or retrognathia and nasal pharyngeal abnormalities, and hypothyroidism and acromegaly. **(p. 694)**

17.8 Narcolepsy is another sleep disorder associated with great functional impairment. All of the following are features of narcolepsy *except*

A. Excessive daytime sleepiness.
B. Cataplexy.
C. Sleep paralysis.
D. Hypnopompic hallucinations.
E. Hypnagogic hallucinations.

The correct response is option D.

Hypnopompic hallucinations are not characteristic of narcolepsy.

Narcolepsy is characterized by the presence of four symptoms: excessive daytime sleepiness, cataplexy, sleep paralysis, and hypnagogic hallucinations. **(p. 695)**

17.9 The parasomnias are a class of behavior disorders occurring during sleep. Which of the following is considered to be the most common parasomnia?

A. Nocturnal seizures.
B. Sleepwalking.
C. Sleep terrors.
D. Nightmares.
E. Bruxism.

The correct response is option A.

According to current estimates based on data from the national cooperative study of patients seen in sleep disorders centers (Coleman et al. 1982), the most commonly encountered parasomnias are those secondary to nocturnal seizure activity (33.7%).

After that, the most common conditions currently classified as parasomnias are sleepwalking, sleep terrors, sleep-related enuresis, nightmares, familial sleep paralysis, head banging, and bruxism. **(pp. 687 [Figure 17–6C], 698)**

17.10 A patient suddenly screams or cries, abruptly sits up in bed, appears to be intensely fearful, is unresponsive to external stimuli, and vocalizes incoherently. Later, the patient is amnestic for the episode. The most likely diagnosis is

A. Nightmare.
B. Rapid eye movement (REM) sleep behavior disorder.
C. Sleepwalking.
D. Rhythmic movement disorder.
E. Sleep terror.

The correct response is option E.

Sleep terror is characterized by sudden arousal with intense fearfulness, which may begin with a piercing scream or cry. Autonomic and behavioral correlates of fright typically mark the experience. An individual experiencing a sleep terror usually sits up in bed, is unresponsive to stimuli, and if awakened is confused or disoriented. Vocalizations may occur but they are usually incoherent. Notwithstanding the intensity of these events, amnesia for the episodes usually occurs. Like sleepwalking, these episodes usually arise from slow-wave sleep. Unlike nightmares, in which an elaborate dream sequence unfolds, sleep terrors may be devoid of images or may contain only fragments of very brief, frighteningly vivid or sometimes static images. **(p. 698)**

17.11 Rapid eye movement (REM) sleep behavior disorder is a rare condition in which patients "act out their dreams" due to a failure of REM-associated atonia. This condition has been associated with use of all the following medication classes or agents *except*

A. Serotonin antagonists.
B. Tricyclic antidepressants (TCAs).
C. Monoamine oxidase inhibitors (MAOIs).
D. Venlafaxine.
E. Serotonin agonists.

The correct response is option A.

Serotonin antagonists are not associated with REM sleep behavior disorder.

Biperiden, TCAs, MAOIs, caffeine, venlafaxine, selegiline, and serotonin agonists can precipitate or exacerbate REM sleep behavior disorder, which can also occur during withdrawal from alcohol, meprobamate, pentazocine, and nitrazepam. **(p. 700)**

Reference

Coleman RM, Roffwarg HP, Kennedy SJ, et al: Sleep-wake disorders based on a polysomnographic diagnosis. A national cooperative study. JAMA 247:997–1003, 1982

CHAPTER 18

Neuropsychiatric Aspects of Cerebrovascular Disorders

Select the single best response for each question.

18.1 Among the following, which is the least common type of cerebrovascular disease?

A. Ruptured aneurysm.
B. Intracerebral hemorrhage.
C. Lacunae.
D. Cerebral embolism.
E. Atherosclerotic thrombosis.

The correct response is option A.

Ruptured aneurysms and arterial venous malformations are the fifth most common types of cerebrovascular disease, after thrombosis, embolism, lacunae, and intracerebral hemorrhage.

Atherosclerotic thrombosis, which accounts for approximately one-third of all incidents of stroke, is often the result of a dynamic interaction between hypertension and the atherosclerotic deposition of hyaline-lipid material in the walls of peripheral, coronary, and cerebral arteries. Risk factors for atherosclerosis include hyperlipidemia, diabetes mellitus, hypertension, and cigarette smoking. Cerebral embolism, which also accounts for approximately one-third of all strokes, is usually caused by a fragment breaking away from a thrombus within the heart and traveling up the carotid artery. Of all the types of stroke, those due to cerebral embolism develop most rapidly. Lacunae, which account for nearly one-fifth of strokes, are the result of occlusion of small penetrating cerebral arteries. Lacunar infarctions may be so small as to produce no recognizable deficits or, depending on their location, may be associated with pure motor or sensory deficits. Intracerebral hemorrhage (ICH), the fourth most frequent cause of stroke, can be the result of hypertension, rupture of saccular aneurysms or arteriovenous malformations, a variety of hemorrhagic disorders of assorted etiologies, and trauma. The prognosis for ICH is grave, with 70%–75% of patients dying within 30 days. **(pp. 707–708)**

18.2 The onset of major depression within the first 2 months following a stroke is most common when the stroke affects which of the following brain regions?

A. Right anterior.
B. Right posterior.
C. Left anterior.
D. Left posterior.
E. Bilateral posterior.

The correct response is option C.

Robinson (2003) found that the lateralized effect of left anterior stroke lesions on both major and minor depression was a phenomenon of the acute poststroke period (i.e., within 2 months following stroke). Left anterior lesions were more than twice as likely as left posterior lesions to produce depression. Similarly, a comparison of left and right anterior lesions showed a similar twofold increase in depression with the left-sided lesions. **(pp. 715–716; Table 18–3)**

18.3 In comparisons of patients with poststroke depression with poststroke patients who did not develop depression, investigators found which of the following to increase the risk of depression following stroke?

A. Older age.
B. Greater subcortical atrophy.
C. Female sex.
D. Lower socioeconomic status.
E. Less education.

The correct response is option B.

Patients with poststroke major depression had significantly more subcortical atrophy ($P < 0.05$), as measured both by the ratio of third ventricle to brain and by the ratio of lateral ventricle to brain (Starkstein et al. 1988). Patients who did and who did not develop depression did not differ on a number of important demographic variables, including age, gender, socioeconomic status, and education. The groups also did not differ on family or personal history of psychiatric disorders or neurological deficits. **(pp. 716–717)**

18.4 Although poststroke mania occurs much less frequently than does poststroke depression, secondary mania may sometimes develop following a stroke. Poststroke mania is most frequently associated with damage to which of the following brain regions?

A. Left anterior frontal.
B. Left posterior temporal.
C. Left occipital.
D. Bilateral anterior.
E. Right hemisphere.

The correct response is option E.

Poststroke patients who develop mania have a significantly greater frequency of lesions in the right hemisphere, compared with poststroke patients who develop depression or no mood disturbance. The right hemisphere lesions that lead to mania tend to be in specific right hemisphere structures that have connections to the limbic system. The right basotemporal cortex appears to be particularly important, in that direct lesions as well as distant hypometabolic effects of this cortical region are frequently associated with secondary mania. **(p. 723)**

18.5 Which of the following statements concerning poststroke anxiety disorder is *true*?

A. Few patients with generalized anxiety disorder (GAD) meet criteria for major depression.
B. Late-onset GAD is associated with a history of psychiatric disorder.
C. Depression with anxiety is associated with right cortical lesions.
D. Over time, the strongest correlates of GAD are an absence of social contacts outside the family and dependence on others to perform activities of daily living (ADLs).
E. GAD has not been associated with cortical atrophy.

The correct response is option D.

Astrom (1996) examined 71 acute stroke patients for anxiety disorder and followed these patients over 3 years. The strongest correlates of GAD were an absence of social contacts outside the family and dependence on others to perform primary ADLs. These factors were significantly more common in the GAD than in the non-GAD population at 3 months and at 1, 2, and 3 years after stroke. At the 3-year follow-up, GAD was associated with both cortical atrophy and greater subcortical atrophy. In a study by Starkstein et al. (1990), 23 of 47 patients with poststroke major depression met criteria for GAD. Castillo et al. (1993, 1995) found that 78 patients (27%) of a group of 288 patients hospitalized with an acute stroke met DSM-III-R (American Psychiatric Association 1987) criteria for GAD (excluding the 6-month duration criteria). Most patients with GAD also had major or minor depression (i.e., 58 of 78 patients with GAD also had depression). Depression plus anxiety was associated with left cortical lesions, whereas anxiety alone was associated with right hemisphere lesions. Early-onset but not late-onset GAD was associated with a history of psychiatric disorder, including alcohol abuse, and early-onset anxiety had a duration of 1.5 months, whereas delayed-onset GAD had a mean duration of 3 months. **(p. 725)**

18.6 Which of the following statements concerning patients with catastrophic reactions to stroke is *false*?

A. Patients have a higher frequency of familial history of psychiatric disorders.
B. Patients have higher rates of major depression.
C. Patients are more likely to be aphasic.
D. Patients more commonly have a personal history of psychiatric disorders.
E. Patients have a higher frequency of basal ganglia lesions.

The correct response is option C.

Catastrophic reaction is not significantly more frequent among aphasic than among nonaphasic patients. This finding does not support the contention that catastrophic reactions are an understandable psychological response of "frustrated" aphasic patients.

Patients with catastrophic reactions were found to have a significantly higher frequency of familial and personal history of psychiatric disorders (mostly major depression) than patients without catastrophic reactions. Patients with catastrophic reactions also have higher rates of major depression and a significantly higher frequency of lesions involving the basal ganglia. One may conclude that catastrophic reaction may have a neurophysiological underpinning, rather than being just a behavioral response of patients confronted with their limitations. **(pp. 727–728)**

References

American Psychiatric Association: Diagnostic and Statistical Manual of Mental Disorders, 3rd Edition, Revised. Washington, DC, American Psychiatric Association, 1987

Astrom M: Generalized anxiety disorder in stroke patients: a 3-year longitudinal study. Stroke 27:270–275, 1996

Castillo CS, Starkstein SE, Fedoroff JP, et al: Generalized anxiety disorder after stroke. J Nerv Ment Dis 181:100–106, 1993

Castillo CS, Schultz SK, Robinson RG: Clinical correlates of early-onset and late-onset poststroke generalized anxiety. Am J Psychiatry 152:1174–1179, 1995

Robinson RG: The controversy over post-stroke depression and lesion location. Psychiatric Times 20:39–40, 2003

Starkstein SE, Robinson RG, Price TR: Comparison of patients with and without poststroke major depression matched for size and location of lesion. Arch Gen Psychiatry 45:247–252, 1988

Starkstein SE, Cohen BS, Fedoroff P, et al: Relationship between anxiety disorders and depressive disorders in patients with cerebrovascular injury. Arch Gen Psychiatry 47:246–251, 1990

C H A P T E R 1 9

Neuropsychiatric Aspects of Brain Tumors

Select the single best response for each question.

19.1 The most common type of primary brain tumor is

A. Meningioma.
B. Glioma.
C. Pituitary adenoma.
D. Medulloblastoma.
E. Neurilemmoma.

The correct response is option B.

Gliomas are the most common (40%–55%) type of primary brain tumors, followed by meningiomas (10%–20%), pituitary adenomas (10%), neurilemmomas (5%–8%), medulloblastomas (5%), and miscellaneous primary tumors (5%). **(p. 735 [Table 19–1])**

19.2 The most common primary site for a central nervous system (CNS) metastatic tumor is

A. Lung.
B. Breast.
C. Kidney.
D. Gastrointestinal tract.
E. Skin.

The correct response is option A.

The most common primary site for a CNS metastatic tumor is the lung (35%–45%), followed by the breast (10%–20%), the kidney and the gastrointestinal tract (5%–10%), and the skin (i.e., melanoma) (2%–5%). **(p. 736 [Table 19–2])**

19.3 Tumors of the frontal lobe may be associated with the "dorsolateral prefrontal syndrome." All of the following are features of this syndrome *except*

A. "Pseudopsychopathic" behavior.
B. Apathy.
C. Indifference.
D. Psychomotor retardation.
E. Poor initiation of tasks.

The correct response is option A.

Pseudopsychopathic behavior—a term referring to personality changes manifesting as irritability, lability, poor judgment, and lack of insight—is not associated with the dorsolateral prefrontal syndrome; rather, this presentation characterizes the orbitofrontal syndrome.

Patients with dorsolateral prefrontal syndrome often present with apathy, indifference, and psychomotor retardation. Cognitively, they have difficulty initiating or persisting in behavioral activities and show problems with sustained attention and/or sequencing, and they may demonstrate perseverative behavior. These deficits may not be especially apparent on standard intellectual or neuropsychological assessments, but they usually become apparent with more specific tests of executive functioning, such as the Wisconsin Card Sorting Test. Patients with this syndrome have been described as being *pseudodepressed*, because the apathy, aspontaneity, and abulia with which they often present resemble the classic symptoms of major depression. **(p. 741)**

19.4 Although tumors of the temporal lobes may present with symptoms similar to classic schizophrenia, certain phenomenological differences have been noted between the two conditions. Symptoms more typically associated with temporal lobe tumors than with classic schizophrenia include all of the following *except*

A. Visual hallucinations.
B. Olfactory hallucinations.
C. Tactile hallucinations.
D. "Spells" and dreamlike episodes.
E. Flat or inappropriate affect.

The correct response is option E.

Flat or inappropriate affect, a classic symptom of schizophrenia, is not seen in patients with temporal lobe tumors; rather, these patients often exhibit a broad range of affect and appropriate interpersonal behavior.

The psychotic symptoms manifested by temporal lobe tumor patients are somewhat atypical for classic schizophrenia and include episodic mood swings with suicidal ideation or attempts and visual, olfactory, and tactile hallucinations, as well as the auditory hallucinations more typically seen in schizophrenic patients. Patients with schizophrenia-like psychoses due to temporal lobe disease also often report having "spells" or dreamlike episodes, as well as "staring" behavior or "dazed feelings." **(p. 743)**

19.5 Tumors of the nondominant parietal lobe may produce the constellation of symptoms called Gerstmann's syndrome. Which of the following is *not* a feature of this syndrome?

A. Hemi-neglect.
B. Dysgraphia.
C. Acalculia.
D. Finger agnosia.
E. Left–right confusion.

The correct response is option A.

Hemi-neglect is not a feature of Gerstmann's syndrome.

Gerstmann's syndrome is characterized by dysgraphia, acalculia, finger agnosia, and right–left confusion and often affects reading and spelling. **(p. 744)**

19.6 Bitemporal hemianopsia, optic atrophy, and diabetes insipidus are symptoms associated with tumors of which region?

A. Pineal.
B. Cerebellum.
C. Basal ganglia.
D. Pituitary.
E. Occipital lobes.

The correct response is option D.

Clinical signs and symptoms associated with pituitary tumors include bitemporal hemianopsia, optic atrophy, hypopituitarism, and diabetes insipidus.

Loss of upward gaze, also know as Parinaud's syndrome, is a symptom of pineal tumors. Tumors of the cerebellum are marked by ipsilateral hypotonia, ataxia, dysmetria, intention tremor, and nystagmus toward the side of the tumor. Symptoms of basal ganglia tumors are contralateral choreoathetosis, dystonia, rigidity, motor perseveration, and parkinsonian tremor. Occipital lobe tumors present with partial sensory seizures with visual phenomena, homonymous hemianopsia, alexia, agraphia, prosopagnosia, color agnosia, and construction apraxia. **(p. 748 [Table 19–3])**

19.7 Systemic findings that should trigger increased suspicion for brain tumor in patients with behavioral symptoms include all of the following *except*

A. Nonfocal neurological signs.
B. Seizures.
C. Headaches.
D. Sensory changes.
E. Nausea and vomiting.

The correct response is option A.

Nonfocal neurological signs are not indicative of a brain tumor.

Psychiatric and behavioral symptoms suggestive of a brain tumor include seizures; new-onset headaches; nausea and vomiting; visual changes such as loss or diminution of vision, visual field defects, or diplopia; auditory changes such as tinnitus or hearing loss, especially when unilateral, and vertigo; and other focal neurological signs and symptoms, such as localized weakness, localized sensory loss, paresthesias or dysesthesias, ataxia, and incoordination. **(p. 747)**

19.8 In treatment of depression in a brain tumor patient who is at risk of seizures, which of the following agents should be avoided?

A. Fluoxetine.
B. Venlafaxine.
C. Maprotiline.
D. Sertraline.
E. Paroxetine.

The correct response is option C.

Maprotiline and bupropion appear to have the greatest seizure-inducing potential among the antidepressants.

Clinical and animal studies report variable effects of tricyclic antidepressants on seizure threshold, and the evidence is unclear as to which antidepressants carry the smallest overall risk, although the selective serotonin reuptake inhibitors in general have been reported to have a low likelihood of precipitating seizures. **(pp. 754, 755)**

CHAPTER 20

Neuropsychiatric Aspects of Human Immunodeficiency Virus Infection of the Central Nervous System

Select the single best response for each question.

20.1 Which of the following statements concerning the epidemiology of acquired immunodeficiency syndrome (AIDS) and human immunodeficiency virus (HIV) infection is *false*?

A. In the United States, approximately 950,000 persons are living with HIV.
B. Worldwide, there are 38 million people living with HIV.
C. In the United States, the annual rate of diagnosis of HIV/AIDS has increased approximately 4% over the 2000–2003 time period.
D. Up to 30% of HIV-infected individuals may be expected to develop HIV-1-associated dementia during the course of the infection.
E. In the United States, approximately 930,000 persons have a diagnosis of AIDS.

The correct response is option C.

U.S. surveillance reports from 2000 to 2003 indicate that the overall annual rate of diagnosis of HIV/AIDS remained stable over this time period, with an increase of 3% in the annual rates of males and a decrease of 3.7% in the annual rates of females. Of these HIV cases, up to 30% may be expected to develop HIV-1-associated dementia.

According to the Centers for Disease Control and Prevention *HIV/AIDS Surveillance Report* through 2003, approximately 950,000 persons in the United States are living with HIV and are largely asymptomatic. Another estimated 929,985 have a diagnosis of AIDS. Worldwide, there are 38 million people living with HIV. **(p. 766)**

20.2 The most common opportunistic infection in AIDS, which may present as a focal or diffuse cognitive or affective disturbance, is

A. Syphilis.
B. *Toxoplasma gondii*.
C. Cytomegalovirus.
D. *Cryptococcus neoformans*.
E. Progressive multifocal leukoencephalopathy.

The correct response is option B.

Toxoplasma gondii is perhaps the most common opportunistic infection in AIDS and may present as a focal or diffuse cognitive or affective disturbance. Clinically, toxoplasmosis symptoms include malaise, confusion, lethargy, headache, fever, and focal deficits.

Syphilis occurs as a concurrent central nervous system (CNS) infection, and its diagnosis is problematic. It can be asymptomatic, and other causes of meningitis can obscure the picture. Cytomegalovirus is commonly seen in the CNS of AIDS patients and may produce encephalitis, retinitis, and peripheral neuropathies and demyelination. *Cryptococcus neoformans* presents principally as meningitis, with headache, altered mental status, nuchal rigidity, fever, and nausea and vomiting. Definitive diagnosis is based on analysis of cerebrospinal fluid. Progressive multifocal leukoencephalopathy is another viral infection producing personality and behavioral changes and cognitive impairment, with or without sensorimotor impairments. **(pp. 769–770)**

20.3 According to American Academy of Neurology (AAN) criteria for HIV-1-associated minor cognitive/motor disorder, diagnostic cognitive/motor/behavioral dysfunctions include all of the following *except*

A. Impaired attention/concentration.
B. Impaired memory.
C. Slowed movements.
D. Incoordination.
E. Disturbance of consciousness.

The correct response is option E.

Disturbance of consciousness is not among the AAN criteria for HIV-1-associated minor cognitive/motor disorder (Janssen et al. 1991). Specific cognitive/motor/behavioral dysfunctions listed in criterion A are impaired attention/concentration, mental slowing, impaired memory, slowed movements, and incoordination, as well as personality change, irritability, or emotional lability. These cognitive/motor dysfunctions must be documented by neurological examination or neuropsychological testing. Furthermore, the dysfunction in cognitive/motor/behavioral abilities must cause mild impairment of work-related activities or activities of daily living. **(p. 774 [Table 20–2])**

20.4 Which of the following statements concerning the treatment of delirium in HIV patients is *true*?

A. In neuroleptic treatment of HIV delirium, initial doses may need to be lower than those used in other medically ill populations.
B. Neuroleptic malignant syndrome is the most common adverse side effect of intravenous haloperidol.
C. Use of intravenous haloperidol to treat delirium is approved by the U.S. Food and Drug Administration.
D. Doses of intravenous medications should not be increased to high levels.
E. Adverse effects of haloperidol in HIV-infected patients are much less frequent if the patient has another coexisting mental disorder due to a general medical condition.

The correct response is option A.

In treatment of HIV delirium, neuroleptic medications should be initiated at the lowest dosage that achieves the desired clinical effects. HIV-positive patients are often more sensitive to neuroleptics and may require lower doses than do other medically ill patients with delirium.

Neuroleptic malignant syndrome is rare in HIV patients. Administration of intravenous haloperidol is still considered investigational. Dosages of intravenous medications may need to be increased to high levels, under watchful observation, to control severe agitation. Adverse effects of haloperidol in HIV-infected patients are mainly extrapyramidal and are significantly more likely if the patient has another coexisting mental disorder due to a general medical condition. **(pp. 781–782)**

20.5 Which of the following antidepressants should be avoided in treatment of HIV/AIDS depression?

A. Escitalopram.
B. Mirtazapine.
C. Citalopram.
D. Nefazodone.
E. Bupropion.

The correct response is option D.

Nefazodone should be avoided in the treatment of depression in HIV/AIDS patients, because of its affinity for cytochrome P450 (leading to drug–drug interactions) and its propensity to cause hepatotoxicity.

Citalopram and escitalopram should be considered first-line selective serotonin reuptake inhibitors in the management of HIV-related depression. Mirtazapine may be particularly useful in patients with HIV-1 infection with severe dyssomnia associated with weight loss. Bupropion has both noradrenergic and dopaminergic effects and has been used effectively in HIV/AIDS patients with depression; however, it has been associated with seizures and should be used cautiously (or avoided altogether) in patients with neurological disease. **(p. 783)**

References

Centers for Disease Control and Prevention: HIV/AIDS Surveillance Report. Atlanta, GA, Centers for Disease Control and Prevention, 2003

Janssen RS, Cornblath DR, Epstein LG, and the Working Group of the American Academy of Neurology AIDS Task Force: Nomenclature and research case definitions for neurologic manifestations of human immunodeficiency virus-type 1 (HIV-1) infection. Neurology 41:778–785, 1991

CHAPTER 21

Neuropsychiatric Aspects of Endocrine Disorders

Select the single best response for each question.

21.1 Cross-sectional and prospective studies have revealed significant cognitive deficits in patients with diabetes mellitus. Which of the following statements concerning diabetes-associated cognitive impairment/decline is *false*?

A. Diabetes increases the risk of both vascular dementia and Alzheimer's disease in older patients.
B. Children with insulin-dependent diabetes mellitus (IDDM) (type I diabetes) suffer from cognitive impairment, with poor metabolic control as a risk factor.
C. Executive function is particularly at risk in IDDM children with disease onset before 4 years of age.
D. Hypoglycemia impairs cognition irreversibly.
E. Greater than 15 years' duration of diabetes increases the risk of cognitive decline.

The correct response is option D.

Hypoglycemia acutely impairs cognition, but the impairment is corrected upon return to a euglycemic state.

Several studies have revealed significant cognitive deficits occurring in patients with both type I and type II diabetes mellitus. These deficits range from cognitive impairment and decline among all age groups, to vascular dementia and Alzheimer's disease among the older population. There continues to be concern that children and adolescents diagnosed with IDDM are at higher risk for more immediate cognitive impairment. In a study by Northam et al. (2001) in which 90 children with IDDM were followed over 6 years and compared with a community control group, the children with diabetes "performed more poorly than control subjects on measures of intelligence, attention, processing speed, long-term memory, and executive skills. Attention, processing speed, and executive skills were particularly affected in children with onset of disease before 4 years of age, whereas severe hypoglycemia was associated with lower verbal and full-scale intelligence quotient scores" (p. 1541). The presence of diabetes for a duration greater than 15 years considerably increased the risk of major cognitive decline. **(pp. 800, 801)**

21.2 The symptoms of hypoglycemia in diabetic patients have significant behavioral components. For classification purposes, these symptoms are divided into the "autonomic" and "neuroglycopenic" symptoms. Which of the following is considered to be an "autonomic" symptom?

A. Confusion.
B. Tremor.
C. Lethargy.
D. Speech changes.
E. Incoordination.

The correct response is option B.

Tremor, diaphoresis, palpitations, and hunger are autonomic symptoms, whereas confusion, lethargy, speech and behavioral changes, and incoordination are neuroglycopenic symptoms. **(p. 803)**

21.3 The metabolic syndrome associated with non-insulin-dependent diabetes mellitus (NIDDM) (type II diabetes) is also seen with the use of atypical antipsychotic agents. All of the following are characteristic of this metabolic syndrome *except*

A. Insulin resistance.
B. Abdominal obesity.
C. Hypertension.
D. Decreased insulin production.
E. Dyslipidemia.

The correct response is option D.

Decreased insulin production is not characteristic of NIDDM, whereas insulin resistance, abdominal obesity, hypertension, and dyslipidemia are well-defined components of the metabolic syndrome. **(p. 804)**

21.4 Treatment of depression in diabetic patients is crucial to promote metabolic stability and to enhance life functioning. All of the following statements are true *except*

A. Remission of depression is achieved in only a small percentage of cases over 5 years.
B. Depression relapses in diabetic patients occur at a rate of one episode per year.
C. Response rates to antidepressant treatment in diabetic patients are only 50% of response rates in nondiabetic patients.
D. Monoamine oxidase inhibitors (MAOIs) exacerbate hypoglycemia and are associated with weight gain.
E. Anticholinergic side effects of some antidepressants can worsen diabetes-related gastroparesis.

The correct response is option C.

Rates of successful treatment of depression among diabetic individuals are similar to those among the general population.

Once depression in diabetic patients has been treated effectively, remission of symptoms is sustained only 10% of the time over the subsequent 5 years. Depression relapses occur at a rate of approximately one per year. MAOIs tend to exacerbate hypoglycemia and are associated with significant weight gain. The decrease in bowel motility caused by anticholinergic medications may worsen underlying diabetes-related gastroparesis or constipation. **(pp. 805–806)**

21.5 Hypothyroidism is an endocrinological illness of great interest to the neuropsychiatrist and serves as a convenient model for psychiatric symptoms due to systemic illness. Which of the following is the most commonly reported psychiatric symptom in hypothyroidism?

A. Depression.
B. Bipolar disorder.
C. Psychotic disorders.
D. Anxiety disorders.
E. Cognitive disorders.

The correct response is option E.

Disturbances in cognition are the most commonly reported psychiatric symptom in hypothyroidism, seen in nearly 50% of cases. The severity of the disturbance varies from mild subjective cognitive slowing to severe delirium and encephalopathy. **(pp. 807, 809 [Figure 21–1])**

21.6 Hypothyroidism is classified on a grading scale correlated to clinical and laboratory abnormalities. "Subclinical hypothyroidism," which is associated with depression and is characterized by elevated thyroid-stimulating hormone (TSH), normal levels of thyroid hormones, and an exaggerated TSH response to thyrotropin-releasing hormone (TRH), would be classified as grade ___.

A. I.
B. II.
C. III.
D. IV.
E. V.

The correct response is option B.

Grade II hypothyroidism is defined by elevated TSH levels with normal plasma levels of thyroid hormones.

Grade I hypothyroidism, or classic primary hypothyroidism, is defined by low levels of circulating thyroid hormones, triiodothyronine (T_3), and thyroxine (T_4), and an elevated TSH concentration accompanied by clinical symptoms. Grade III hypothyroidism is characterized by an exaggerated TSH response to TRH in the presence of normal basal TSH, T_3, and T_4 levels. Grade IV hypothyroidism, or symptomless autoimmune thyroiditis, is characterized by the abnormal presence of antithyroid antibodies in the serum with normal circulating basal TSH, T_3, and T_4 levels and normal TRH stimulation test results. **(p. 810)**

21.7 As with hypothyroidism, hyperthyroidism is associated with significant degrees of psychiatric comorbidity. Which of the following is the most common psychiatric manifestation of hyperthyroidism?

A. Psychosis.
B. Cognitive disturbance.
C. Mania.
D. Major depression.
E. Anxiety.

The correct response is option D.

In this chapter's summary of the case literature and studies involving unselected hyperthyroid patients, major depression was the most common psychiatric manifestation of hyperthyroidism, occurring in approximately 28% of patients.

Although anxiety is cited as one of the cardinal features of hyperthyroidism, it appeared in only 13% of unselected patients in whom anxiety symptoms were sought. The prevalence of cognitive disturbance in thyrotoxicosis was 7.4%, considerably less than that observed in hypothyroidism. Mania or hypomania secondary to hyperthyroidism was distinctly uncommon, occurring in only 2.1% of unselected cases. Psychosis was likewise an uncommon manifestation of thyrotoxicosis, occurring in only 2.1% of patients. **(pp. 811, 812 [Table 21–3; Figure 21–2], 813)**

21.8 Corticosteroid-induced psychiatric symptoms are a serious consequence of long-term steroid therapy. Which of the following agents is *not* a recommended pharmacotherapeutic strategy for managing these symptoms?

A. Lamotrigine.
B. Lithium.
C. Tricyclic antidepressants (TCAs).
D. Valproic acid.
E. Olanzapine.

The correct response is option C.

TCAs have been shown to exacerbate corticosteroid-induced psychiatric symptoms and are therefore not a treatment option.

Lithium, lamotrigine, valproic acid, and olanzapine have all been used to prevent steroid-induced psychiatric symptoms. **(p. 817)**

21.9 Hypoparathyroidism is associated with a wide range of psychiatric symptoms. Which of the following psychiatric disorders is the most prevalent in hypoparathyroidism?

A. Mood disorders.
B. Anxiety disorders.
C. Cognitive disorders.
D. Psychotic disorders.
E. Dissociative disorders.

The correct response is option C.

Numerous psychiatric symptoms have been reported in hypoparathyroidism, including irritability and affective, anxiety, psychotic, and cognitive disorders. Cognitive disorders are the most frequently encountered. Dissociative disorders are not common in hypoparathyroidism. **(p. 821)**

Reference

Northam EA, Anderson PJ, Jacobs R, et al: Neuropsychological profiles of children with type 1 diabetes 6 years after disease onset. Diabetes Care 24:1541–1546, 2001

CHAPTER 22

Neuropsychiatric Aspects of Poisons and Toxins

Select the single best response for each question.

22.1 Which of the following solvents produces peripheral neuropathy as its most common adverse side effect?

A. Ethylbenzene.
B. Ethylene glycol.
C. Carbon tetrachloride.
D. Methyl-*n*-butyl ketone.
E. Methanol.

The correct response is option D.

Methyl-*n*-butyl ketone produces peripheral neuropathy as its most common adverse effect. Ethylbenzene produces headache, irritability, and fatigue. Ethylene glycol produces fatigue, personality change, and depression. Carbon tetrachloride produces lethargy and confusion. Methanol produces visual toxicity, loss of visual acuity, and parkinsonian syndrome. **(p. 838 [Table 22–3])**

22.2 High plasma aluminum concentrations have been associated with various neuropsychiatric symptoms. Which of the following plasma aluminum levels has been associated with incoordination, intention tremor, cognitive deficits, loss of balance, and memory defects?

A. <10 µg/L.
B. 10–60 µg/L.
C. 61–100 µg/L.
D. 101–200 µg/L.
E. >200 µg/L.

The correct response is option E.

Plasma aluminum concentration higher than 200 µg/L has been associated with incoordination, intention tremor, cognitive deficits, loss of balance, and memory loss.

Plasma aluminum concentrations less than 10 µg/L usually produce no symptoms. Levels between 10 and 60 µg/L are associated with objective changes in neurophysiological and neuropsychological measures. Levels between 61 and 100 µg/L are associated with subtle mental changes such as directional disorientation and personality changes. Finally, levels between 101 and 200 µg/L have been shown to produce impairment in memory, abstract reasoning, and depression. **(p. 840 [Table 22–7])**

22.3 Common sources of lead exposure include all of the following *except*

A. Pesticides.
B. Battery production.
C. Printing.
D. Soldering.
E. Welding.

The correct response is option A.

Use of pesticides is not associated with lead exposure.

Common sources of lead exposure are battery production, brass and bronze work, cable making/splicing, chemical operations, glassworks, ammunition production, jewelry production, lead smelting, metal casting and refining, paint production, pigment production, pipe cutting, pottery manufacturing, printing, soldering, stained-glass manufacturing, and welding. **(p. 842 [Table 22–9])**

22.4 In a study conducted by Min (1986), which of the following psychiatric symptoms was found in the majority of patients who exhibited the delayed syndrome associated with carbon monoxide intoxication?

A. Depressed mood.
B. Delusions.
C. Echolalia.
D. Apathy.
E. Elated mood.

The correct response is option D.

Apathy, disorientation, amnesia, hypokinesia, mutism, irritability or distractibility, apraxia, and bizarre behaviors were found in more than 60% of patients who suffered from carbon monoxide intoxication. Depressed mood was noted in only 15% of patients with carbon monoxide poisoning, delusions in 12%, echolalia in 2%, and elated mood in 2% (Min 1986). **(p. 847 [Table 22–11])**

22.5 Which of the following herbal preparations is frequently used as a sedative?

A. Cola nut.
B. Kava.
C. Valerian.
D. Yohimbine.
E. Peyote.

The correct response is option C.

Valerian is frequently used as a sedative.

Cola nut is a stimulant. Kava and peyote are hallucinogens, and yohimbine is a mild hallucinogen. **(pp. 857–858 [Table 22–13])**

22.6 Nerve agents are particularly potent organophosphates used for chemical warfare. What is their mechanism of action?

A. They act at the membrane level, particularly on sodium channels.
B. They inactivate the enzyme acetylcholinesterase.
C. They produce a marked loss of neurons in the hippocampus and amygdaloid nucleus.
D. They combine with hemoglobin in the blood.
E. They produce a primary axonal neuropathy.

The correct response is option B.

Nerve agents have the capacity to inactivate the enzyme acetylcholinesterase.

Pyrethroids act at the membrane level, particularly on sodium channels. Domoic acid produces a marked loss of neurons in the hippocampus and amygdaloid nucleus. Carbon monoxide combines with hemoglobin in the blood to form carboxyhemoglobin. Ethylene oxide produces a primary axonal neuropathy. **(pp. 847, 848, 851, 855, 864–865)**

Reference

Min SK: A brain syndrome associated with delayed neuropsychiatric sequelae following acute carbon monoxide intoxication. Acta Psychiatr Scand 73:80–86, 1986

CHAPTER 23

Neuropsychiatric Aspects of Ethanol and Other Chemical Dependencies

Select the single best response for each question.

23.1 Opiate dependence mechanisms at the level of the locus coeruleus (LC) help explain the physiological effects of these substances. Which of the following statements concerning the LC's role in opiate dependence/withdrawal is *false?*

A. Overactivation of the LC is necessary and sufficient to produce behavioral signs of opiate withdrawal.
B. The action of the α_1-adrenergic blocker clonidine mimics the effects of morphine on the LC.
C. Extrinsic activation of the LC involves excitatory glutamatergic input from the nucleus paragigantocellularis.
D. Intrinsic activation of the LC includes adaptations in opioid receptor–coupled signal transduction.
E. The LC contains the major noradrenergic nucleus in the brain.

The correct response is option B.

Clonidine, which has effects similar to those of morphine on neurons of the locus coeruleus, is an α_2-adrenergic agonist, not an α_1-adrenergic blocker. **(p. 886)**

23.2 Which of the following statements regarding the intrinsic locus coeruleus (LC) mechanism of opiate dependence is *true?*

A. Acute opiate inhibition of the LC neurons involves inhibition of the G protein–activated inward-rectifying K^+ (GIRK) channel.
B. Acute opiate inhibition of the LC neurons involves activation of inward Na^+ current.
C. Only GIRK channel effects are mediated by pertussis toxin–sensitive G proteins.
D. G proteins inhibit the GIRK channel via an indirect mechanism.
E. G protein–mediated inhibition of cyclic adenosine monophosphate (cAMP) formation influences the Na^+ current.

The correct response is option E.

G protein–mediated inhibition of cAMP formation inhibits the Na^+ current.

Acute opiate inhibition of the LC neurons involves activation of the GIRK channel and inhibition of the inward Na^+ current. GIRK and Na^+ channels are both mediated via pertussis toxin–sensitive G proteins. **(pp. 886, 887 [Figure 23–4])**

23.3 The mesolimbic dopamine system is involved in the reinforcing properties of several substances of abuse. However, one group of abused substances produces behavioral reinforcement independently of the dopamine system, by acting on receptors in the nucleus accumbens and other regions. Which of the following substances produces reinforcement independent of the dopamine system?

A. Opiates.
B. Psychostimulants.
C. Cannabinoids.
D. Ethanol.
E. Nicotine.

The correct response is option A.

Opiates, such as heroin and morphine, produce reinforcement independently of the dopamine system by acting directly on opioid receptors in the nucleus accumbens and other brain regions. The other substances act by dopamine-dependent mechanisms. **(p. 889)**

23.4 "Cross-priming," wherein dosing of one group of substances leads to increased use of another class of abusable drugs, is thought to be mediated by the mesolimbic dopamine system. Cross-priming has been clearly demonstrated for which two groups of drugs?

A. Cannabinoids and psychostimulants.
B. Cannabinoids and alcohol.
C. Nicotine and hallucinogens.
D. Opiates and alcohol.
E. Opiates and psychostimulants.

The correct response is option E.

Cross-priming has been demonstrated only for opiates and psychostimulants. **(pp. 889–890)**

23.5 "Stress-induced" relapse into drug-seeking behavior has been studied in both animals and human subjects. Which of the following statements is *true*?

A. In animals, stress-related heroin relapse requires physiological dependence.
B. Stress-induced dopamine release in the nucleus accumbens correlates with relapse into heroin-seeking behavior.
C. Stress-induced relapse into drug use is completely attenuated with dopamine antagonists.
D. Stress attenuates release of corticotropin-releasing factor (CRF), which correlates with opiate relapse.
E. Corticosterone infusion blocks drug-seeking relapse.

The correct response is option B.

Stress-induced dopamine release in the nucleus accumbens correlates temporally with relapse to heroin-seeking behavior.

Stress-induced relapse to heroin-seeking behavior is equally effective whether animals are physically dependent on heroin or not. Stress-induced relapse is partially attenuated by pretreatment with dopamine antagonists. Stress stimulates release of CRF. Corticosterone can induce relapse to cocaine-seeking behavior. **(p. 891)**

23.6 What is the presumed neurochemical action of hallucinogens?

A. Stimulation of monoamine release.
B. Antagonist at *N*-methyl-D-aspartate (NMDA) glutamate receptors.
C. Antagonism of 5-hydroxytryptamine 2A (5-HT_{2A}) serotonin receptors.
D. Partial agonism at 5-hydroxytryptamine 1A (5-HT_{1A}) serotonin receptors.
E. Partial agonism at 5-HT_{2A} serotonin receptors.

The correct response is option E.

Hallucinogens cause partial agonism at 5-HT_{2A} serotonin receptors.

Amphetamine stimulates monoamine release. Phencyclidine causes antagonism in the NMDA glutamate receptors. **(p. 883 [Table 23–1])**

23.7 "Altered physiological state that causes a withdrawal syndrome when drug taking ceases" is the definition of which of the following?

A. Tolerance.
B. Sensitization.
C. Dependence.
D. Reinforcement.
E. Addiction.

The correct response is option C.

Dependence is an altered physiological state that causes a withdrawal syndrome when drug taking ceases.

Reduced drug effect at constant dose is called *tolerance. Sensitization* is increased drug effect at constant dose. *Reinforcement* is a stimulus action that increases a behavioral response. *Addiction* is compulsive drug use despite adverse consequences or loss of control over drug use. **(p. 899 ["Highlights for the Clinician"])**

23.8 Mechanisms of dopamine-induced relapse depend on an understanding of different dopamine receptor subtypes and their effects. Which of the following statements is *true?*

A. $Dopamine_1$ (D_1)–like (D_1 and D_5) receptors are negatively coupled to adenylyl cyclase.
B. $Dopamine_2$ (D_2)–like (D_2, D_3, and D_4) receptors are positively coupled to adenylyl cyclase.
C. In the nucleus accumbens (NAc), activation of D_1-like receptors produces relapse to cocaine use in rats.
D. D_1-like receptors are responsible for priming effects in the NAc.
E. D_1-like receptor activation abolishes the ability of cocaine to induce relapse.

The correct response is option E.

D_1-like receptor activation completely abolishes the ability of cocaine to induce relapse.

D_1-like (D_1 and D_5) receptors are positively coupled to adenylyl cyclase activity, whereas the D_2-like (D_2, D_3, and D_4) receptors are either negatively coupled or have no detectable effect on the enzyme. Activation of D_2-like, but not of D_1-like, dopamine receptors induces a profound and prolonged relapse to cocaine-seeking behavior in rats. D_2-like receptors are primarily involved in inducing drug-seeking behavior by priming stimuli that release dopamine in the NAc. **(p. 892)**

23.9 Which of the following substances causes decreased dendritic arborizations and decreased terminal dendritic spine density in the nucleus accumbens (NAc)?

A. Cocaine.
B. Amphetamine.
C. Nicotine.
D. Morphine.
E. None of the above.

The correct response is option D.

Long-term morphine administration causes decreased terminal dendritic spine density in the NAc. Long-term administration of cocaine, amphetamine, or nicotine increases the dendritic arborization of the medium spiny neurons of the NAc as well as the density of their terminal dendritic spines. **(pp. 896–897)**

CHAPTER 24

Neuropsychiatric Aspects of Dementias Associated With Motor Dysfunction

Select the single best response for each question.

24.1 Which of the following degenerative dementias with motor involvement is autosomal recessively inherited?

A. Huntington's disease.
B. Parkinson's disease.
C. Friedreich's ataxia.
D. Frontotemporal dementia.
E. Wilson's disease.

The correct response is option E.

Wilson's disease is autosomal recessively inherited.

Huntington's and Parkinson's diseases, Friedreich's ataxia, and frontotemporal dementia are all autosomal dominantly transmitted. **(p. 909 [Table 24–2])**

24.2 All of the following psychiatric disorders have been described in the literature as common comorbid conditions in Huntington's disease *except*

A. Schizophreniform disorder.
B. Intermittent explosive disorder.
C. Major depression.
D. Obsessive-compulsive disorder.
E. Bipolar disorder.

The correct response is option D.

Obsessive-compulsive disorder is infrequently comorbid with Huntington's disease.

Schizophreniform disorder was once thought to be the most common psychiatric manifestation of Huntington's disease but probably is more common in advanced cases. Studies using explicit diagnostic criteria and standardized assessments suggest that intermittent explosive disorder and affective disorders (especially unipolar depression , but also bipolar disorder) are the most prevalent psychiatric disorders in Huntington's disease. **(p. 913)**

24.3 The psychiatric disorder most commonly found in patients with Parkinson's disease is

A. Psychosis.
B. Affective disorder.
C. Obsessive-compulsive disorder.
D. Generalized anxiety disorder.
E. Intermittent explosive disorder.

The correct response is option B.

Affective disorder is the most common psychiatric disturbance in Parkinson's disease, with an estimated incidence of from 20% to 90%. Depression frequently goes unrecognized, and when it is recognized, it is often untreated or undertreated. Medications trigger the vast majority of episodes of psychosis in Parkinson's disease. Celesia and Wanamaker (1972) observed psychotic episodes in 12% of their 153 patients. Most of these episodes were caused by antiparkinsonian medications and occurred in patients who were cognitively impaired. Intermittent explosive disorder is more frequently seen in Huntington's disease than in Parkinson's disease. Obsessive-compulsive disorder and generalized anxiety disorder are infrequently seen in Parkinson's disease. **(pp. 916–917)**

24.4 All of the following are clinical characteristics of diffuse Lewy body disease *except*

A. Dementia.
B. Attentional impairment.
C. Apathy.
D. Parkinsonism.
E. Fluctuations in cognitive functioning.

The correct response is option C.

Apathy is not a clinical characteristic of diffuse Lewy body disease.

Key clinical characteristics of diffuse Lewy body disease include dementia, attentional impairment, parkinsonism, fluctuations in cognitive functioning, visuospatial difficulties, and persistent, well-formed visual hallucinations. **(pp. 918, 919 [Table 24–5])**

24.5 Which of the following clinical findings is helpful in distinguishing progressive supranuclear palsy (PSP) from Parkinson's disease?

A. Vertical eye movement abnormalities.
B. Dementia.
C. Stable gait.
D. Postural stability.
E. Axial parkinsonism with tremor.

The correct response is option A.

PSP may be distinguished from Parkinson's disease and other progressively degenerative motor disorders by the following constellation of clinical findings: axial parkinsonism without tremor, unstable gait with postural instability, and vertical eye movement abnormalities without alien limb movements. The earliest eye movement abnormalities include loss of vertical saccade velocity. With disease progression, pursuit eye movements are also impaired. Unlike parkinsonism in Parkinson's disease or cortical–basal ganglionic degeneration, parkinsonism in PSP is almost always symmetrical in severity. Many patients with PSP have no noticeable dementia, and dementia is often not severe early in the course of the disease. **(pp. 919–920; Table 24–6)**

24.6 In Wilson's disease, which brain structure degenerates in association with abnormalities in liver function?

A. Thalamus.
B. Hippocampus.
C. Amygdala.
D. Basal ganglia.
E. Corpus callosum.

The correct response is option D.

In Wilson's disease, also called hepatolenticular degeneration, the basal ganglia degenerate in association with abnormalities in liver function. **(p. 924)**

Reference

Celesia GG, Wanamaker WM: Psychiatric disturbances in Parkinson's disease. Diseases of the Nervous System 33:577–583, 1972

CHAPTER 25

Neuropsychiatric Aspects of Alzheimer's Disease and Other Dementing Illnesses

Select the single best response for each question.

25.1 The Neuropsychiatric Inventory (NPI) completed by the caregivers of patients with mild cognitive impairment (MCI) can quantify the psychiatric comorbidity of this particular cognitive disorder. All of the following symptoms are common in MCI *except*

A. Euphoria.
B. Dysphoria.
C. Apathy.
D. Irritability.
E. Anxiety.

The correct response is option A.

Euphoria is a relatively uncommon symptom of MCI, as are hallucinations, delusions, abnormal motor behavior, and disinhibition. **(pp. 936–937; Figure 25–1)**

25.2 Alzheimer's disease is the most common dementia in the United States. As this disease progresses, a series of neurobehavioral symptoms are encountered. Which of the following symptoms develop after significant disease progression, rather than early in the course of the disease?

A. Deficient verbal and visual encoding.
B. Impaired delayed recall.
C. Concrete thinking.
D. Mild anomia.
E. Transcortical sensory aphasia.

The correct response is option E.

Transcortical sensory aphasia (with relatively preserved syntax and phonological abilities) is not an early symptom of Alzheimer's disease; rather, it develops later, as the disease progresses.

Symptoms seen early in the disease course include deficient verbal and visual encoding, impaired delayed recall, concrete thinking, and mild anomia. Patients may have trouble operating a vehicle and/or managing their finances. They also may suffer from deficient emotional processing, as manifested in difficulty with interpretation of facial expression and speech prosody. **(pp. 937–938)**

25.3 Alzheimer's disease is associated with many behavioral symptoms, all of which can contribute significantly to functional impairment. Which of the following is the most common neuropsychiatric symptom in Alzheimer's disease?

A. Depressed mood.
B. Anxiety.
C. Apathy.
D. Irritability.
E. Psychosis.

The correct response is option C.

Apathy, consisting of loss of interest, motivation, volition, enjoyment, spontaneity, and emotional behavior, is the most common neuropsychiatric symptom in Alzheimer's disease, affecting 42% of patients with mild, 80% of those with moderate, and 92% of those with advanced Alzheimer's disease. **(p. 939; Figure 25–3)**

25.4 The neuropathology of Alzheimer's disease features neuritic plaques. These plaques are deposited in different areas of cortical tissue in a progressive way. What is the site of the first deposition of plaques?

A. Frontal association cortex.
B. Parietal cortex.
C. Perirhinal cortex.
D. Temporo-occipital association cortex.
E. Entorhinal cortex.

The correct response is option D.

The plaques first appear in the temporo-occipital association regions, then spread to the entorhinal and perirhinal, the parietal, and later the frontal association cortices. **(p. 941; Figure 25–5)**

25.5 Which medication for Alzheimer's disease blocks butyrylcholinesterase as well as acetylcholinesterase?

A. Memantine.
B. Rivastigmine.
C. Galantamine.
D. Tacrine.
E. Donepezil.

The correct response is option B.

Rivastigmine blocks butyrylcholinesterase as well as acetylcholinesterase.

The acetylcholinesterase inhibitors donepezil, galantamine, and rivastigmine were the first pharmaceuticals approved by the U.S. Food and Drug Administration for treatment of Alzheimer's disease. Rivastigmine and galantamine have additional mechanisms of action: rivastigmine blocks butyrylcholinesterase, and galantamine is an allosteric modulator of the nicotinic presynaptic receptors. Memantine, a weak *N*-methyl-D-aspartate (NMDA) receptor blocker, is approved for treatment of moderate to severe Alzheimer's disease. **(pp. 942–943)**

25.6 In 2005, the Expert Consensus Panel for Dementia published guidelines for treatment of psychiatric comorbidity in dementia. Which of the following was recommended as a first-line treatment for insomnia in dementia?

A. Risperidone.
B. Quetiapine.
C. Olanzapine.
D. Clonazepam.
E. Mirtazapine.

The correct response is option B.

The panel recommended trazodone or quetiapine both as short-term and as long-term first-line agents for insomnia (Alexopoulos et al. 2005). Other recommended agents were zolpidem, risperidone, mirtazapine, and olanzapine. Clonazepam was not recommended. **(pp. 944, 945)**

25.7 Dementia with Lewy bodies (DLB) can be distinguished from Alzheimer's disease (AD) on clinical grounds. Cognitive symptoms that are more common and severe in DLB than AD include all of the following *except*

A. Attentional deficits.
B. Visual hallucinations.
C. Cognitive fluctuations.
D. Fluctuating alertness with episodes of delirium.
E. Memory impairment.

The correct response is option E.

Cognitive decline in DLB is somewhat different from that observed in AD. Memory impairment is less severe in DLB than in AD, but attention and visuospatial and visuoperceptual functions can be severely affected early in the disease course. Whereas in AD cognitive fluctuations are minor, in DLB they are profound, and large variability in cognitive performance on attention and executive tasks has been described. DLB patients often have fluctuating alertness and clear-cut episodes of delirium. **(p. 945)**

25.8 Which of the following atypical antipsychotics is the preferred agent for treatment of hallucinations in dementia with Lewy bodies (DLB)?

A. Clozapine.
B. Olanzapine.
C. Quetiapine.
D. Risperidone.
E. None of the above.

The correct response is option E.

Neuroleptic use is *contraindicated* in DLB because of the extreme risk of severe side effects and death. Adverse reactions to antipsychotics reported in this patient population include sedation, confusion, severe parkinsonism with extreme rigidity and immobility, and neuroleptic malignant syndrome. **(pp. 946, 948)**

25.9 Which of the following is *not* a feature of primary progressive aphasia?

A. Early prominent language impairment.
B. Dysfluent and agrammatic speech.
C. Early loss of language comprehension.
D. Anomia.
E. Phonemic paraphasic errors.

The correct response is option C.

Language comprehension (except for grammatically complex linguistic constructs) is preserved until late in the disease course of primary progressive aphasia.

Primary progressive aphasia is a type of frontotemporal dementia characterized by early prominent language impairment. The patient's speech is dysfluent, effortful, and agrammatic, with pronounced anomia and phonemic paraphasic errors. **(p. 949)**

25.10 Vascular dementia (VaD) of the multi-infarct type is another common dementia. The constellation of cognitive symptoms in VaD suggests a subcortical pattern of deficits. All of the following deficits are typical of VaD *except*

A. Psychomotor slowing.
B. Dysexecutive symptoms.
C. Poor encoding of memory with adequate retrieval.
D. Impaired attention.
E. Poor set shifting.

The correct response is option C.

Relative to Alzheimer's disease, vascular dementia is characterized by a retrieval as opposed to an encoding pattern of memory deficit.

Neuropsychological deficits in VaD primarily involve psychomotor slowing and dysexecutive problems. Declines in attention, processing speed, and set shifting are readily observed. Language difficulties are common; dysarthria may be present, along with shorter phrase length and simplified vocabulary and syntax. **(p. 953)**

25.11 Delusional misidentification syndromes occur mostly later in the disease course of dementia. Which of the following syndromes involves a conviction that a physical location has been duplicated?

A. Capgras' syndrome.
B. Fregoli's syndrome.
C. Foley's syndrome.
D. Doppelganger.
E. Reduplicative paramnesia.

The correct response is option E.

Reduplicative paramnesia is the belief that a physical location (e.g., one's home) has been duplicated.

Capgras' syndrome is the belief that others, usually close relatives, have been replaced by impostors. Fregoli's syndrome is the belief that strangers have been replaced by familiar people. Foley's syndrome is the delusion that one's image in the mirror is that of another person. Doppelganger is the belief that one has a double. **(p. 940, 941 [Table 25–3])**

Reference

Alexopoulos GS, Jeste DV, Chung H, et al: The expert consensus guideline series. Treatment of dementia and its behavioral disturbances. Introduction: methods, commentary, and summary. Postgrad Med (Special Report):6–22, 2005

CHAPTER 26

Neuropsychiatric Aspects of Schizophrenia

Select the single best response for each question.

26.1 In a long-term follow-up study of patients with schizophrenia (the Vermont study), many of these patients, after 10 years of follow-up and approximately 15–20 years of illness, showed

A. A marked deterioration in mental functioning.
B. No psychotic symptoms.
C. A poor level of overall functioning, especially those over 50 years of age.
D. A deteriorating long-term course.
E. Little heterogeneity in outcome.

The correct response is option B.

More than half of the individuals in the Vermont study (Harding et al. 1987a, 1987b) had no psychotic symptoms after 10 years of follow-up, and they were found to have considerable heterogeneity in outcome in later life. After the initial deteriorating years, the later course of the illness settles at a low, but flat, plateau. Surprisingly, symptoms often improve after age 50 years, and most individuals with schizophrenia have a "good" level of functioning in their later lives. **(p. 972)**

26.2 Which of the following candidate genes implicated in schizophrenia has also been associated with velocardiofacial syndrome?

A. Dystrobrevin binding protein-1 (*DTNBP1*).
B. Neuregulin-1 (*NRG1*).
C. Catechol-O-methyltransferase (COMT).
D. Disrupted-in-schizophrenia-1 and -2 (*DISC1* and *DISC2*).
E. Metabotropic glutamate receptor-3 (*GRM3*).

The correct response is option C.

CO*MT* maps to 22q11, the deletion of which produces velocardiofacial syndrome, a disease associated with a high incidence of psychosis. **(pp. 973, 974)**

26.3 Magnetic resonance imaging (MRI) studies of the brains of patients with schizophrenia have revealed a volume decrease in all of the following brain structures *except*

A. Hippocampus.
B. Amygdala.
C. Parahippocampal gyrus.
D. Superior temporal gyrus.
E. Caudate nucleus.

The correct response is option E.

A volume decrease of the caudate nucleus has not been revealed in MRI studies of schizophrenic patients.

MRI studies have consistently revealed a volume decrease in the medial temporal cortical structures, hippocampus, amygdala, and parahippocampal gyrus. The volume of the superior temporal gyrus has also been reported as being reduced in schizophrenia, and the magnitude of the reduction has been correlated with the presence of hallucinations and with electrophysiological changes in the patients. **(p. 977)**

26.4 A number of neurotransmitters have been implicated in schizophrenia. Phencyclidine (PCP) and ketamine cause a schizophrenic-like reaction in humans and affect which of the following neurotransmitters?

A. Dopamine.
B. Serotonin.
C. Nicotine.
D. Glutamine.
E. Acetylcholine.

The correct response is option D.

The glutamate system has become a focus of study in schizophrenia because of its ubiquitous and prominent location in the central nervous system and because the antiglutamatergic drugs PCP and ketamine cause a schizophrenic-like reaction in humans. **(p. 980)**

26.5 The MATRICS (measurement and treatment research to improve cognition in schizophrenia) program was developed to identify potential molecular targets to treat cognitive deficits in schizophrenia (Geyer and Tamminga 2004). The molecular targets identified as having the greatest promise to improve cognition include all of the following *except*

A. Dopamine$_1$ (D_1) receptor.
B. Dopamine$_2$ (D_2) receptor.
C. α_7 Nicotinic receptor.
D. Muscarinic receptor.
E. *N*-methyl-D-aspartate (NMDA) receptor.

The correct response is option B.

The D_2 receptor has not been identified as a molecular target to treat cognitive deficits in schizophrenia.

The D_1 receptor, the α_7 nicotinic receptor, the muscarinic receptor, the 5-hydroxytryptamine 1A (5-HT_{1A}) and 5-HT_{2A} receptors, the noradrenergic receptors, and the NMDA receptor are believed to have the greatest promise as potential molecular targets to treat cognitive deficits in schizophrenia. **(p. 986)**

26.6 Positron emission tomography (PET) scanning in hallucinating persons with schizophrenia has provided clues to the anatomic structures that may be involved in a "psychosis neural circuit." The proposed psychosis circuit consists of all of the following structures *except*

A. Amygdala.
B. Medial prefrontal cortex.
C. Thalamus.
D. Anterior hippocampus.
E. Anterior cingulate.

The correct response is option A.

The amygdala is not involved in the proposed "psychosis neural circuit"; rather, it is implicated in the emotional processing of schizophrenia and is believed to be involved in a "negative affect neural circuit."

PET scanning in hallucinating persons with schizophrenia has found activations in the medial prefrontal cortex, left superior temporal gyrus, right medial temporal gyrus, left hippocampus/parahippocampal region, thalamus, putamen, and cingulate. These studies provide clues to the anatomic structures that may be involved in a "psychosis neural circuit." The proposed psychosis circuit consists of the anterior hippocampus, anterior cingulate, medial prefrontal cortex, thalamus, ventral pallidum, striatum, and substantia nigra/ventral tegmental area. **(pp. 987, 988; Figure 26–4)**

References

Geyer MA, Tamminga CA: Measurement and treatment research to improve cognition in schizophrenia: neuropharmacological aspects. Psychopharmacology (Berl) 174:1–2, 2004

Harding CM, Brooks GW, Ashikaga T, et al: The Vermont longitudinal study of persons with severe mental illness, I: methodology, study sample, and overall status 32 years later. Am J Psychiatry 144:718–726, 1987a

Harding CM, Brooks GW, Ashikaga T, et al: The Vermont longitudinal study of persons with severe mental illness, II: long-term outcome of subjects who retrospectively met DSM-III criteria for schizophrenia. Am J Psychiatry 144:727–735, 1987b

C H A P T E R 2 7

Neuropsychiatric Aspects of Mood Disorders

Select the single best response for each question.

27.1 Specific types of cognitive deficits are seen in mood disorders. All of the following cognitive impairments are common in depressed patients *except*

A. Slowed thought process.
B. Impaired attention.
C. Impaired concentration.
D. Language impairment.
E. Executive function impairment.

The correct response is option D.

Specific impairments in language, perception, and spatial abilities are not usually seen in patients with mood disorders (except as a secondary consequence of poor attention, motivation, or organizational abilities).

Cognitive deficits in mood disorders are typically of mild to moderate severity but can become quite severe in prolonged or intractable depression. The cognitive abnormalities typically seen in depressed patients include slowed thought processes, impaired attention and concentration, and impaired executive functioning (planning, organization, short-term memory). Manic patients also show impaired executive functioning (including disinhibition and impulsivity) and poor concentration and attention. **(p. 1006)**

27.2 The neurochemical changes that occur in depression can affect several neurotransmitter systems. Depression is associated with all of the following neurochemical alterations *except*

A. Lower levels of cerebrospinal fluid (CSF) serotonin metabolites.
B. Decreased serotonin transporter binding.
C. Serotonin receptor abnormalities.
D. Decreased CSF homovanillic acid.
E. Increased dopamine transporter activity.

The correct response is option E.

Various studies have suggested that dopamine transporter activity may be *reduced,* not increased, in patients with depression.

Depressed patients show lower CSF levels of serotonin metabolites, decreased serotonin transporter binding, and abnormalities in serotonin receptors. CSF concentrations of homovanillic acid are also reduced in depression. **(pp. 1007, 1008)**

27.3 The neurobiology of depression as currently modeled involves several cortical and subcortical structures. All of the following cortical structures are thought to have a major role in depression *except*

A. Prefrontal cortex.
B. Anterior cingulate cortex.
C. Subgenual cingulate cortex.
D. Medial temporal cortex.
E. Occipital cortex.

The correct response is option E.

The occipital cortex does not have a role in depression. The functional neuroanatomy of mood disorders involves a diverse set of brain structures, including the prefrontal cortex, anterior cingulate cortex, subgenual cingulate cortex, medial temporal cortex, and parietal cortex. **(p. 1011)**

27.4 The effect of depression on sleep patterns offers clues to understanding the neurobiology of depression. Which is the best-studied and most reproducible sleep electroencephalography (EEG) finding in depressed patients?

A. Reduced rapid eye movement (REM) latency.
B. Prolonged sleep latency.
C. Decreased slow-wave sleep.
D. Increased time in REM sleep.
E. Decreased time in non-REM sleep.

The correct response is option A.

Reduced REM latency is the best-studied and most reproducible sleep-related electroencephalography finding in depressed patients, and this abnormality is reversed by most antidepressants.

Sleep abnormalities in depression include prolonged sleep latency, decreased slow-wave sleep, and reduced REM latency, with disturbances in the relative time spent in both REM and non-REM sleep. **(p. 1014)**

27.5 In the neural network model of depression presented in the chapter, distinct neural systems are associated with specific functions (and therefore associated with underlying symptom clusters). Cognitive, psychomotor, and sensory processing are associated with all of the following structures *except*

A. Amygdala.
B. Dorsal prefrontal cortex.
C. Dorsal anterior cingulate cortex.
D. Parietal cortex.
E. Hippocampus.

The correct response is option A.

The amygdala is not associated with the cognitive, psychomotor, and sensorimotor processing; rather, it is one of the brain regions involved in more covert/masked cognitive-emotional processing.

Cognitive, psychomotor, and sensorimotor processing are associated with dorsal prefrontal, dorsal anterior cingulate, parietal and posterior cingulate cortices, and hippocampus. Medial frontal, orbitofrontal, and perigenual anterior cingulate cortices are associated with overt cognitive processing of emotional stimuli, including salience, reward value, and self-relevance. More covert or masked cognitive-emotional processing is associated with medial temporal and subcortical regions, including the amygdala, ventral basal ganglia, and midbrain structures and nuclei. **(pp. 1016–1017; Figure 27–4)**

27.6 Correctly diagnosing a mood disorder in neuropsychiatric patients can be difficult, because symptoms of the neurological illness may mimic or mask the symptoms of mood disturbance. Mood symptoms less likely to be independently associated with the underlying neurological illness than with a primary mood disorder include all of the following *except*

A. Apathy.
B. Mood disturbance with consonant affect.
C. Anhedonia.
D. Excessive guilt.
E. Suicidality.

The correct response is option A.

Apathy (a decreased drive to engage in self-directed activity) commonly occurs in the absence of depression in Parkinson's disease, Alzheimer's dementia, and some types of traumatic brain injury.

Anhedonia (a decreased ability to experience pleasure), on the other hand, is more specific to primary depressive disorder, as also are excessive guilt and suicidality. Mood and affective states associated with primary mood disorders tend to be straightforward, with mood and affect typically corresponding. By contrast, patients with neuropsychiatric disease often present with mood dissociated from affect. **(pp. 1004–1007)**

CHAPTER 28

Neuropsychiatric Aspects of Anxiety Disorders

Select the single best response for each question.

28.1 Various neuroanatomical models have been proposed for selected anxiety disorders. Which anxiety disorder is believed to be associated with increased activity in the ventromedial cortico-striatal-thalamic-cortical (CSTC) circuit?

A. Generalized anxiety disorder.
B. Obsessive-compulsive disorder (OCD).
C. Panic disorder.
D. Posttraumatic stress disorder.
E. Social anxiety disorder.

The correct response is option B.

Current neuroanatomical models of OCD emphasize the role of CSTC circuits. There is growing realization of the importance of various CSTC loops in a range of behavioral disorders, especially OCD. This model of OCD was first suggested by early findings of an association between neurological lesions of the striatum and OCD symptoms. **(pp. 1026, 1029, 1030 [Figure 28–3])**

28.2 Neuroanatomical models of panic disorder emphasize the involvement of a number of brain structures and pathways. Which brain structure is believed to play a central role in conditioned fear and anxiety?

A. Thalamus.
B. Caudate.
C. Locus coeruleus.
D. Amygdala.
E. Periaqueductal gray.

The correct response is option D.

Current neuroanatomical models of panic emphasize the extended amygdala, which is thought to play a central role in conditioned fear and anxiety; the hippocampus, which is thought crucial for conditioning to the context of the fear; and efferent tracts from the amygdala to the hypothalamus and brain stem structures, which mediate many of the symptoms of panic. **(p. 1032; Figure 28–4)**

28.3 Many brain structures are involved in fear and anxiety. Which of the following structures has the highest concentration of noradrenergic-producing neurons in the brain?

A. Thalamus.
B. Hypothalamus.
C. Locus coeruleus.
D. Amygdala.
E. Periaqueductal gray.

The correct response is option C.

The locus coeruleus, which contains the highest concentration of noradrenergic-producing neurons in the brain, plays a key role in fear and anxiety, with both electrical or pharmacological stimulation resulting in fear responses. Several clinical studies of panic disorder provide support for the role of the locus coeruleus in panic. **(pp. 1032–1033)**

28.4 Features of current neuroanatomical models of posttraumatic stress disorder (PTSD) include all of the following *except*

A. The amygdalothalamic pathways are involved in the rapid, automatic processing of incoming information.
B. There is hyperactivation of the amygdala.
C. The hippocampus is involved in remembering the context of traumatic memories.
D. The amygdala sends afferents to the hypothalamus and brain stem nuclei.
E. There is increased activity in certain frontal cortical areas such as Broca's area.

The correct response is option E.

In PTSD, there is decreased activity in certain frontal cortical areas such as Broca's area, consistent with the decreased verbalization during processing of trauma, and with the ability to override automatic amygdala processing. The amygdalothalamic pathways are involved in the rapid, automatic processing of incoming information in PTSD. Also in PTSD, there is believed to be hyperactivation of the amygdala, which in turn sends afferents to the regions involved in anxiety response (especially the hypothalamus and brain stem nuclei). The hippocampus is involved in remembering the context of traumatic memories. **(p. 1034; Figure 28–5)**

28.5 In a study examining the role of various neurochemical circuits in social anxiety disorder, investigators concluded that patients with social anxiety disorder may exhibit selective supersensitivity of which of the following circuits?

A. Serotonergic.
B. Dopaminergic.
C. Nicotinic.
D. Noradrenergic.
E. Cholinergic.

The correct response is option A.

A range of evidence supports the role of serotonergic circuits in social phobia. In a pharmacological probe study performed with agents that affect the serotonergic (fenfluramine), dopaminergic (levodopa), and noradrenergic (clonidine) systems, the only positive finding was an augmented cortisol response to fenfluramine administration in patients with social phobia (Tancer et al. 1994). The dopaminergic system may be involved in social anxiety but in the context of decreased cerebrospinal fluid dopamine levels or differences in dopamine$_2$ (D_2) striated density. Nicotinic and cholinergic circuits in social anxiety disorder have not been studied. **(pp. 1035–1036)**

Reference

Tancer ME, Mailman RB, Stein MB, et al: Neuroendocrine responsivity to monoaminergic system probes in generalized social phobia. Anxiety 1:216–223, 1994

CHAPTER 29

Neuropsychiatric Disorders of Childhood and Adolescence

Select the single best response for each question.

29.1 The emergence of lateralization and hemispheric asymmetry are important to neurobehavioral development. All of the following statements are true *except*

A. Lateralization is largely established by age 5 years.
B. Differential development of the two hemispheres in early growth is due to delayed myelination of the corpus callosum.
C. In early development, the left hemisphere develops more rapidly than the right, due to its usual dominance.
D. The right hemisphere accelerates its development between the ages of 3 and 6 years.
E. Gray matter density tends to be greater in the right posterior temporal regions than the left.

The correct response is option C.

During the first few months of development, the right hemisphere develops more rapidly than the left. However, by age 5–6 months, dendritic growth in the left hemisphere surpasses that in the right hemisphere and continues at a rapid pace for the next 2 years. Between ages 3 and 6 years, the right hemisphere accelerates in its development and helps provide the prosodic components of language that flower between ages 5 and 6. Lateralization of the brain is largely established before 5 years of age and emerges through a multistage process that begins in utero. **(p. 1048)**

29.2 Psychiatric comorbidity in attention-deficit/hyperactivity disorder (ADHD) often complicates this already difficult-to-manage disorder. Which of the following statements is *true*?

A. Conduct disorder occurs in 20%–40% of ADHD cases.
B. Abused children with both posttraumatic stress disorder (PTSD) and ADHD have the same degree of motor hyperactivity as do children with classic ADHD alone.
C. Thyroid hormone resistance is a common cause of ADHD.
D. A high incidence of ADHD is found with girls, but not boys, with Tourette's syndrome.
E. ADHD-type symptoms may indicate genetic risk in schizophrenia pedigrees.

The correct response is option E.

ADHD-type symptoms may indicate genetic risk in children with a family history of schizophrenia.

Conduct disorder is found in 40%–70% of subjects with ADHD. Abused children with PTSD and ADHD are more active than normal children, but substantially less active than children with classic ADHD. Thyroid hormone resistance is very rare and almost never found in children with ADHD. A high incidence of ADHD is also found in boys with Tourette's syndrome. **(p. 1050)**

29.3 Imaging studies have helped to delineate a constellation of brain regions involved in attention-deficit/hyperactivity disorder (ADHD). Which of the following is the most consistent neuroanatomical finding in ADHD subjects relative to non-ADHD controls?

A. Decreased size of the caudate.
B. Increased size of the frontal cortex.
C. Increased size of the posterior portion of the corpus callosum.
D. Decreased size of the cerebellar vermis.
E. Increased size of the anterior portion of the corpus callosum.

The correct response is option D.

The most consistently documented morphometric difference between ADHD subjects and controls is a reduction in the size of the cerebellar vermis, a midline gray and white matter region that connects left and right cerebellar hemispheres. Interestingly, this is the brain region that shows the greatest degree of growth during the postnatal period. The caudate volume appears to decrease with age in boys without ADHD, presumably as a consequence of pruning, but does not appear to change with age in boys with ADHD. Some studies have documented a decrease in the size of the posterior corpus callosum, while others have reported that the anterior portion of the corpus callosum is reduced in size in boys with ADHD. **(pp. 1051, 1052)**

29.4 Psychostimulant medications remain the cornerstone of attention-deficit/hyperactivity disorder (ADHD) treatment. Common side effects of psychostimulants include all of the following *except*

A. Anorexia.
B. Irritability.
C. Dysphoria.
D. Tics and other stereotypic movements.
E. Insomnia.

The correct response is option D.

Tics and other stereotypic movements are uncommon side effects of psychostimulants.

The side effects most commonly reported with psychostimulant medications are anorexia, stomach-aches, insomnia, and mood changes (irritability, mood lability, dysphoria). **(p. 1056)**

29.5 Tic disorders are often comorbid with obsessive-compulsive disorder (OCD). However, the OCD symptoms in tic disorder patients often differ from the symptoms in patients with classic OCD. All of the following statements are true *except*

A. OCD is seen in approximately 10% of Tourette's syndrome patients.
B. OCD symptoms usually appear 1–2 years before simple tics in these patients.
C. Tic-related OCD has an earlier onset than does classic OCD.
D. Tic-related OCD features more ritualized touching and tapping than does classic OCD.
E. Tic-related OCD has a less favorable response to selective serotonin reuptake inhibitors (SSRIs) and a more favorable response to antipsychotic augmentation compared with classic OCD.

The correct response is option B.

In Tourette's syndrome patients who develop OCD, the symptoms usually appear 5–10 years after the first appearance of simple tics. Tic-related OCD may differ from classic OCD, with an earlier onset; more prominent symptoms of ritualized touching, tapping, and rubbing; a less satisfactory response to SSRIs; and an enhanced response to neuroleptic augmentation. **(p. 1059)**

29.6 Fragile X syndrome, the most common known inherited cause of mental retardation, is often associated with autism-spectrum behaviors. Which of the following symptoms is *not* characteristic of fragile X syndrome?

A. Social withdrawal and reduced caregiver attachment.
B. Gaze avoidance.
C. Hand flapping.
D. Tactile defensiveness.
E. Perseveration.

The correct response is option A.

Social withdrawal and reduced attachment to caregivers are *not* characteristic of fragile X syndrome. Many patients affected by fragile X syndrome show autistic features such as gaze avoidance, hand flapping, tactile defensiveness, and perseveration. **(p. 1064)**

29.7 Prader-Willi syndrome is a genetic form of mental retardation characterized by specific morphological and behavioral abnormalities. Which of the following features is *not* characteristic of this illness?

A. Growth retardation.
B. Precocious sexual development.
C. Obesity.
D. Hyperphagia.
E. Short stature.

The correct response is option B.

Precocious sexual development is not a feature of Prader-Willi syndrome.

Food-related difficulties, including childhood onset of pronounced obesity associated with hyperphagia, are the most striking and widely recognized sequelae of this syndrome. Other characteristic features of Prader-Willi syndrome include infantile hypotonia and poor suck reflex, growth retardation, delayed sexual development, hypogenitalism, short stature, small hands and feet, almond-shaped eyes, strabismus, skin-picking, and low activity levels. **(p. 1066)**

29.8 Seizure disorders in children are a vexing source of neurological and psychiatric symptoms. A childhood seizure that features alterations in consciousness; auras of unpleasant odors, tastes, and sensations; and simple, repetitive, and purposeless automatisms is classified as what type of seizure?

A. Simple partial seizure.
B. Partial sensory seizure.
C. Rolandic epilepsy.
D. Complex partial seizure.
E. Frontal lobe epilepsy.

The correct response is option D.

Complex partial seizures, also known as *psychomotor* or *temporal lobe seizures*, are the most frequent form of focal epilepsy in children and are distinguished from other partial seizures by alterations in consciousness.

Frontal lobe epilepsy is the second most frequent localized form of epilepsy. Initial manifestations of frontal lobe seizures depend on the location of the epileptogenic zone. *Simple partial seizures* may be motor or sensory. A simple partial motor seizure consists of recurrent clonic movements of one part of the body without loss of consciousness. *Partial sensory seizures* consist of paresthesias or pain referred to a single part of the body. They also can spread. In general, partial seizures last 1–2 minutes and are not associated with loss of consciousness. *Rolandic epilepsy* is a benign, inherited focal epileptic disorder of childhood that is the most common form of focal seizure seen in children younger than 15 years of age. **(pp. 1077–1078)**

29.9 Pediatric autoimmune neuropsychiatric disorders associated with streptococcal infection (PANDAS) presents a fascinating model of infectious disease–associated neuropsychiatric illness. The Swedo criteria for PANDAS include all of the following *except*

A. Presence of obsessive-compulsive disorder (OCD) and/or tic disorder.
B. Onset before age 7 years.
C. Episodic course of symptom severity.
D. Association with group A β-hemolytic streptococcal (GABHS) infection.
E. Association with neurological abnormalities.

The correct response is option B.

Onset of PANDAS occurs before puberty, not necessarily before age 7 years.

Swedo et al. (1998), who provided the first characterization of PANDAS, proposed that patients with the syndrome could be identified by the following five criteria: 1) the presence of OCD and/or a tic disorder, 2) age at onset before puberty, 3) episodic course of symptom severity, 4) association with GABHS infection, and 5) association with neurological abnormalities. **(p. 1083)**

Reference

Swedo SE, Leonard HL, Garvey M, et al: Pediatric autoimmune neuropsychiatric disorders associated with streptococcal infections: clinical description of the first 50 cases. Am J Psychiatry 155:264–271, 1998

CHAPTER 30

Intracellular and Intercellular Principles of Pharmacotherapy for Neuropsychiatric Disorders

Select the single best response for each question.

30.1 Which of the following statements concerning glia (astrocytes) is *false*?

A. Glia protect neurons by limiting synaptic levels of glutamate.
B. Glia play a prominent role in recycling and conserving glutamate.
C. Glia possess membrane transporters for glutamate.
D. Glutamate is metabolized to γ-aminobutyric acid (GABA) in the glial cell.
E. Glutamate is involved in opening of specific calcium channels that allow influx of calcium ions into neurons.

The correct response is option D.

Glutamate is metabolized to glutamine, a neuronally inactive substance, not to GABA.

Glutamate and GABA are ubiquitous neurotransmitters in the brain, serving as primarily excitatory and inhibitory neurotransmitters, respectively. Glial cells play a prominent role in recycling and conserving both glutamate and GABA by recapturing them from the synapse, converting them to glutamine, and returning glutamine to the presynaptic neurons for conversion back to the appropriate neurotransmitter. In addition, glia protect neurons by limiting synaptic levels of glutamate. Prominent among glutamate's various cellular influences is the opening of specific calcium channels that allow the influx of calcium ions into neurons. The overstimulation of neurons via this mechanism has been associated with neurotoxicity and neuronal death. Glial cells have been shown to possess membrane transporters or uptake sites for glutamate. **(pp. 1118–1119)**

30.2 Astroglia play a pivotal role in the regulation of brain physiology and neuronal activity via the nitric oxide (NO) pathway. Which of the following is the precursor of NO?

A. Glutamate.
B. γ-Aminobutyric acid (GABA).
C. L-Arginine.
D. Glutamine.
E. Glutamine synthetase.

The correct response is option C.

Astroglia play a pivotal role in the regulation of brain physiology and neuronal activity via the NO pathway. They accumulate and store L-arginine, the precursor of NO, and at least under some circumstances, can accumulate the metabolic precursor of L-arginine and synthesize L-arginine. The L-arginine stored in the astroglia is then available for NO synthesis and modification of neuronal activity, neuronal energy metabolism, and regulation of local blood flow through NO action on epithelial cells lining the microvasculature. **(p. 1121)**

30.3 Chemical transmission requires the presence of several elements to operate effectively. These elements may focus on the presynaptic, synaptic, or postsynaptic portion of the neuron. Which of the following elements is required for chemical transmission at the synaptic level?

A. Enzymes for neurotransmitter synthesis.
B. Coupler proteins.
C. Mechanism for neurotransmitter storage.
D. Neurotransmitter receptors to initiate response.
E. Mechanism for terminating neurotransmitter action.

The correct response is option E.

The element required for chemical transmission at the synaptic level is the mechanism for terminating neurotransmitter action.

Elements required at the presynaptic level are enzymes for neurotransmitter synthesis, a mechanism for neurotransmitter storage, a mechanism for appropriate neurotransmitter release, and neurotransmitter receptors for feedback modification of neurotransmitter release. At the postsynaptic level, chemical transmission requires neurotransmitter receptors to initiate response, coupler proteins, and a mechanism for response involving ion channels/second messenger systems. **(p. 1122; Table 30–2)**

30.4 Which of the following receptor types has seven transmembrane sections of the protein with extracellular and intracellular loops that serve as neurotransmitter binding sites?

A. Receptors that form ion channels.
B. G protein–coupled receptors.
C. Receptors that act on allosteric sites.
D. Steroid transcription factor binding receptors.
E. Receptors that synthesize components of synaptic transmission.

The correct response is option B.

Neuroreceptors can be placed into four broad categories, depending on the mode of action of their physiological response. The most prevalent receptors are those that connect to a second-messenger system through one of a family of proteins referred to as G proteins. This receptor type is characterized by having seven transmembrane sections of the protein with extracellular and intracellular loops that serve as neurotransmitter binding sites and sites for receptor regulation.

A second category of neuroreceptors consists of those receptors that form membrane ion channels or ionophores. Stimulation of receptors in this class opens ion channels specific for sodium, potassium, calcium, and chloride ions. The third class of neuroreceptors consists of receptors that attach to allosteric sites on other neuroreceptors regulating receptor ligand affinities. Examples include the benzodiazepine and associated receptors that modify γ-aminobutyric acid (GABA) receptor activity, as well as the glycine B receptor, associated with the *N*-methyl-D-aspartate (NMDA) subtype of glutamate receptor. The fourth class of neuroreceptors is made up of intraneuronal receptors best characterized by steroid transcription factor binding and the synthesis of various components of synaptic transmission, such as enzymes, receptors, and second-messenger systems. **(p. 1127)**

30.5 At this time, only one known psychotherapeutic agent likely has its mechanism of action in a second-messenger system. This agent is...

A. Lithium.
B. Haloperidol.
C. Chlorpromazine.
D. Carbamazepine.
E. Clozapine.

The correct response is option A.

At present, lithium is the only known psychotherapeutic agent thought to have its mechanism of action in a second-messenger system. Lithium, an agent for treating mania, is well known to block inositol monophosphatase, a critical enzyme in the synthesis of phosphatidylinositol and the subsequent production of inositol-1,4,5-trisphosphate (IP_3). This is a suggested mechanism of lithium's antimanic action, because the influences on IP_3 occur at therapeutic doses. **(pp. 1133–1134)**

30.6 Which of the following statements concerning nitric oxide (NO) is *true*?

A. NO is stored in presynaptic nerve endings.
B. NO interacts with specific receptors.
C. NO's influence is synaptic in nature.
D. NO is not a gas in the central nervous system.
E. NO is synthesized on demand.

The correct response is option E.

NO is synthesized on demand. As a gas, it diffuses rapidly through aqueous and lipid beds; thus, its influence is not synaptic in nature. Unlike other neurotransmitters, NO is not stored and released by specific presynaptic nerve endings, and it does not interact with specific receptors. **(p. 1134)**

30.7 Which of the following neurotransmitter types uses only cyclic adenosine monophosphate (cAMP) as its messenger system?

A. Glycine.
B. Angiotensin.
C. Dopamine.
D. Cortisol.
E. Glutamate.

The correct response is option C.

Dopamine, similar to opioids, uses only cAMP as its messenger system. Angiotensin uses cyclic guanosine monophosphate (cGMP). Glycine uses chloride channels, and cortisol uses modification of neurotransmission elements. Glutamate uses calcium channels as its messenger system. **(p. 1129 [Table 30–3])**

CHAPTER 31

Psychopharmacological Treatments for Patients With Neuropsychiatric Disorders

Select the single best response for each question.

31.1 Depression and apathy are common complications of neuropsychiatric illness and require clinical subtlety in their management. Among the following antidepressant agents, which is most likely to be useful for apathy with depressed mood?

A. Amitriptyline.
B. Selective serotonergic and noradrenergic reuptake inhibitors (SNRIs).
C. Doxepin.
D. Nonselective monoamine oxidase inhibitors (MAOIs).
E. Bupropion.

The correct response is option E.

Strategies involving dopaminergic agents have been useful in treating states of apathy in patients with neuropsychiatric disorders. Recommended medications include bupropion, bromocriptine, amantadine, and stimulants. Tricyclic antidepressants, if used, should be limited to desipramine and nortriptyline, and nonselective MAOIs should be avoided in neuropsychiatric patients. **(pp. 1156–1157)**

31.2 Psychosis complicating neuropsychiatric illness can be seen in a number of syndromes but is generally less common than mood disorders. Which of the following is *least* likely to be associated with psychosis?

A. Stroke.
B. Complex partial seizures.
C. Huntington's disease.
D. Human immunodeficiency virus (HIV) disease.
E. Late-stage Parkinson's disease.

The correct response is option A.

Psychosis is relatively uncommon in stroke and multiple sclerosis and is less common in traumatic brain injury (TBI) and early and middle-phase Parkinson's disease. It is more commonly associated with complex partial epilepsy, Huntington's disease and late-stage Parkinson's disease, HIV infection, limbic encephalitis, multi-infarct and Alzheimer's dementias, and tumors involving the temporal lobe and diencephalon. **(p. 1157)**

31.3 Because of the dopamine-deficient state in Parkinson's disease, management of psychosis in this condition poses a significant risk of exacerbating motor symptoms. This can be mitigated somewhat by judicious use of atypical antipsychotics. Which of the following agents in this class is the most efficacious for psychosis in Parkinson's disease?

A. Risperidone.
B. Olanzapine.
C. Aripiprazole.
D. Ziprasidone.
E. Clozapine.

The correct response is option E.

The only medication with confirmed antipsychotic benefit that does not worsen Parkinson's disease is clozapine, at a dose of less than 50 mg/day. However, a number of side effects and potential adverse reactions limit the use of clozapine. Clozapine is associated with significant weight gain, abnormalities in glucose and cholesterol metabolism, and autonomic reactions (increased salivation, increased heart rate, constipation, hypotension). There is an approximately 1% risk of agranulocytosis with clozapine, necessitating close monitoring of white blood cell counts. **(p. 1162)**

31.4 Mania, depression, and anxiety may be associated with a range of neuropsychiatric illnesses. All of the following statements are true *except*

A. Stroke is rarely associated with mania.
B. Mania is far less common in patients with traumatic brain injury (TBI) than in the general population.
C. Multiple sclerosis patients have a higher risk of mania than the general population.
D. Stroke patients with cortical lesions are more likely to have anxiety and depression than are those with subcortical lesions.
E. HIV patients have a higher risk of mania than the general population.

The correct response is option B.

There is much greater incidence of mania in TBI patients than in the general population. **(p. 1163)**

31.5 Lithium has been reported to have a robust effect on which particular type of mania?

A. Mania associated with human immunodeficiency virus (HIV).
B. Mania associated with traumatic brain injury (TBI).
C. Mania associated with steroid use.
D. Mania associated with Parkinson's disease.
E. Mania associated with multiple sclerosis.

The correct response is option C.

Lithium appears to have a robust effect on steroid-induced mania and agitation. However, because of its proconvulsant effects and its ability to cause or aggravate extrapyramidal side effects, it is not considered a first-line choice for most neuropsychiatric patients. **(p. 1167)**

31.6 β-Adrenergic blockers may be a therapeutic option in agitated states. All of the following statements are true *except*

A. Response may take up to 8 weeks.
B. Both central and peripheral β blockade may contribute to these agents' therapeutic action.
C. Secondary depression is common and often limits the use of β-blockers.
D. β-Blockers are contraindicated in chronic obstructive pulmonary disease (COPD).
E. Dosages of up to 12 mg/kg/day are recommended for propranolol.

The correct response is option C.

Secondary depression due to β-blockers appears to be a rare occurrence, but these medications are contraindicated in patients with asthma, COPD, insulin-dependent diabetes, congestive heart failure, persistent angina, significant peripheral vascular disease, and hyperthyroidism. **(p. 1174)**

31.7 Concerning the use of psychostimulants to treat cognitive impairment, which of the following statements is *false*?

A. Stimulants have been shown to improve neuropsychological testing performance in HIV disease.
B. Stimulants are generally well tolerated in neurological patients.
C. Stimulants may enhance cortical recovery.
D. Stimulants lower the seizure threshold, a major limitation in their utility.
E. Stimulants may increase delusional thought content.

The correct response is option D.

Stimulants do *not* appear to lower the seizure threshold at therapeutic levels. They have been found to improve scores on several neuropsychological tests in patients with HIV disease; they are generally well tolerated in the neurological patient and may even enhance cortical recovery. However, psychostimulants should be used with caution because of their potential to aggravate irritability and delusional thought content. **(p. 1179)**

CHAPTER 32

Psychotherapy for Patients With Neuropsychiatric Disorders

Select the single best response for each question.

32.1 Because patients with neuropsychiatric disorders may exhibit impairments in selected hierarchical capacities, psychiatrists will need to adapt their psychotherapeutic techniques to assist the patient in managing these impairments. By adopting a reassuring manner, avoiding overstimulation, and limiting the time of visit, the psychiatrist will address which capacity that may be impaired?

A. Consciousness.
B. Attention.
C. Retention.
D. Orientation.
E. Recognition.

The correct response is option A.

When consciousness is impaired, the psychiatrist should adopt a reassuring manner, avoid overstimulation, limit the time of the visit, assess the changing tolerance for interventions, and keep affect positive.

When *attention* is impaired, the psychiatrist should eliminate distractions, keep one-on-one contact, speak clearly, and simplify language, using brief syntax. If *retention* is impaired, the psychiatrist should simplify communication, repeat things from time to time, reinforce with writing and diagrams, and identify himself or herself at each visit. When *orientation* is impaired, the psychiatrist would do well to remind the patient of time, place, and person; should keep a calendar and a clock in view; and should visit at the same time each day. When *recognition* is impaired, the psychiatrist should tailor the approach to compensate for specific impairments of any of the many parallel brain processors, from trouble with simple geometric perceptions through facial recognition to more complex perceptual components of relationship. Communication should be adapted to assist and circumvent dysphasic channels. **(pp. 1200, 1201 [Table 32–1])**

32.2 Patients with neuropsychiatric disorders may misidentify others. Eight variant forms of misidentification have been described. What is the appropriate term to describe the form of misidentification in which a patient believes that a familiar person has assumed another bodily form?

A. Capgras' delusions, "Body Snatchers" type.
B. Intermetamorphosis.
C. Fregoli type.
D. Subjective doubles, Capgras type.
E. Reverse subjective doubles, autoscopic type.

The correct response is option C.

In the Fregoli type of misidentification, named for the great Italian actor who was a master of disguised identities, a familiar person has assumed another bodily form.

In Capgras' delusions, "Body Snatchers" type, people are being replaced by identical doubles. In intermetamorphosis, both minds and bodies of people are interchanging. In subjective doubles, Capgras type, unseen doubles, phantom boarders, or deceased persons are felt to be present. In reverse subjective doubles, autoscopic type, the person feels either like an imposter or as if he or she is in the process of being replaced. **(pp. 1202, 1205 [Figure 32–2])**

32.3 Traumatic brain injury results principally from vehicular accidents, falls, acts of violence, and sports injuries. Which population age group is at highest risk of such injury?

A. 0–5 years.
B. 6–14 years.
C. 15–24 years.
D. 25–60 years.
E. 61–74 years.

The correct response is option C.

Traumatic brain injury results principally from vehicular accidents, falls, act of violence, and sports injuries and is more than twice as likely to occur in men as in women. The highest incidence is among persons ages 15–24 years and persons age 75 years or older, with a less striking peak in children age 5 years or younger. **(p. 1207)**

32.4 Traumatic brain injury (TBI) will have a profound effect upon families. Which of the following statements concerning the impact of TBI on families is *true*?

A. Wives and mothers of TBI patients may experience increases in anxiety and social dysfunction, but the symptoms are brief, usually lasting less than 6 months.
B. The physical deficits from TBI are more troubling than the cognitive and affective changes.
C. The father of a TBI patient is the parent most likely to be able to handle stress.
D. Mothers of TBI patients usually assume the role of case managers.
E. When TBI patients are hospitalized, the hospital staff is often a source of support to the family, especially when conflicts arise.

The correct response is option D.

Traumatic brain injury in a family member causes a significant increase in the level of stress within the family. According to Solomon and Scherzer (1991, p. 255), when the brain-injured offspring is discharged from the hospital, it is usually the mother who takes on the role of case manager; among family members, the father is the least likely to be able to tolerate the stress and may abandon the family either physically or psychologically.

Solomon and Scherzer (1991, p. 255) have reported that wives and mothers of TBI patients experience increases in anxiety, social dysfunction, and perceived burden as a function of the severity of the injury, and these symptoms persist at least 1–2 years posttrauma. It is the cognitive and affective changes—rather than the physical deficits—of TBI that are the most troublesome for the family. Hospital staff is often guilty of both condescension and wrongly attributing pathology to the family in order to explain conflicts with the hospital staff. The consequences of such conflict include the alienation of the family, who often represent the last resource of the patient, and the loss of potential allies in the rehabilitation process. **(p. 1210)**

32.5 Which of the following statements concerning treatment considerations in early Parkinson's disease is *true?*

A. During the early phases of the illness, patients should be exposed to patients with advanced stages of the illness so they will know what to expect.
B. The patient's significant other should be referred to as the caregiver.
C. Demands from the patient for secrecy of the diagnosis are often indicative of paranoid ideation.
D. Psychotherapy is of little value in managing tremor and bradykinesia.
E. During the early stages, patients should practice being more facially demonstrative.

The correct response is option E.

Whatever the pharmacological therapy, persons with early Parkinson's disease can benefit from psychotherapy to counter stresses that amplify the tremor and bradykinesia. Patients should be encouraged to compensate for parkinsonian facies by practice in remembering to animate the affect, enunciate clearly and loudly enough, and to restore normal gestural fluency as much as possible.

Early in the illness, the patient should be exposed as little as possible to the most advanced cases in support groups or waiting areas. The patient's significant other should not be referred to as the *caregiver,* because for many people this term conjures up the specter of a complete dependent on their hands in the near future. The term *partner* is preferable. Concealment of the diagnosis may be of the highest priority early in the disorder, depending on the patient's occupation, and demands for secrecy are realistic, not paranoid. **(p. 1222)**

32.6 In managing patients with Huntington's disease, psychiatrists should

A. Participate in denial of transmissibility.
B. Discuss fantasies that the disease is a punishment.
C. Avoid addressing family ambivalence about preserving life in a downhill course.
D. Refrain from pointing out that preservation of recognition may lead to depression.
E. Resist the temptation to interpret blame of the gene-donating parent.

The correct response is option B.

The psychiatrist treating a patient with Huntington's disease should discuss fantasies that the disease is punishment, not participate in the denial of transmissibility, address the family's ambivalence about preserving life in a downhill course, note that preservation of recognition may lead to depression, and interpret the blaming of the gene-donating parent.

In addition, the psychiatrist should help the patient internalize his or her healthy heritage from the affected parent, work with envy and rage against unaffected siblings, understand that ideas of blame and prevention are strategies for control, recognize that movement disorders add disability to dementia, ensure that the family has the aid of physiatrists and nutritionists, and encourage caregivers to pace themselves and take recreation. **(pp. 1229, 1230; Table 32–9)**

Reference

Solomon CR, Scherzer BP: Some guidelines for family therapists working with the traumatically brain injured and their families. Brain Inj 5:253–266, 1991

CHAPTER 33

Cognitive Rehabilitation and Behavior Therapy for Patients With Neuropsychiatric Disorders

Select the single best response for each question.

33.1 Cognitive rehabilitation requires tailoring the therapy to the patient's specific deficits. In the Orientation Remedial Program, all of the following task areas are included *except*

A. Attending and reacting to environmental signals.
B. Timing responses in relation to environmental signals.
C. Being actively vigilant.
D. Estimating time.
E. Responding on the basis of simple rhythms.

The correct response is option E.

Responding on the basis of simple rhythms is not included in the Orientation Remedial Program.

The Orientation Remedial Program, a rehabilitation program designed to improve attention, consists of five separate tasks that are presented by microcomputer and vary in degree of difficulty. They involve training in the following areas: 1) attending and reacting to environmental signals, 2) timing responses in relation to changing environmental cues, 3) being actively vigilant, 4) estimating time, and 5) synchronizing of response with complex rhythms. **(p. 1247)**

33.2 Steps in the "PQRST" method for remembering written information include all of the following *except*

A. **P**review of the information.
B. Form **Q**uestions about the information.
C. **R**ehearse responses.
D. **S**tate questions.
E. **T**est for retention.

The correct response is option C.

R stands for **R**ead the information. **(pp. 1248–1249)**

33.3 Patients with frontal lobe impairments often have different rehabilitative needs than those with temporal lobe deficits. Which of the following symptoms is characteristic of temporal, rather than frontal, lobe symptoms?

A. Heightened interpersonal sensitivity and paranoid ideation.
B. Social disinhibition.
C. Reduced attention.
D. Distractibility.
E. Impaired judgment.

The correct response is option A.

Individuals with temporal lobe dysfunction can show heightened interpersonal sensitivity, which can evolve into frank paranoid ideation. **(p. 1253)**

33.4 Various interventions are used to address dysfunctional behaviors observed in individuals with neurological impairment. A behavioral approach wherein there is reinforcement of a behavior inconsistent with the target problem behavior is called

A. Extinction.
B. Positive reinforcement.
C. Negative reinforcement.
D. Differential reinforcement of other behavior.
E. Antecedent management.

The correct response is option D.

In differential reinforcement of other behavior, the effect of the problem behavior is not addressed. Instead, another behavior that is inconsistent with the target problem behavior is reinforced.

In *positive reinforcement,* a behavior is followed by an environmental consequence that increases the likelihood that the behavior will occur again. In *negative reinforcement,* a behavior is followed by the removal of a negative or aversive environmental condition. When the reliable relation between a specific behavior and an environmental consequence is removed, the behavioral effect is to reduce the target behavior to a near-zero level of occurrence, a process called *extinction.* Antecedent management involves identifying and attempting to restructure events that lead to undesirable behavior. **(p. 1255)**